The International Libr...

THE NEURAL BASIS OF
THOUGHT

Founded by C. K. Ogden

The International Library of Psychology

PHYSIOLOGICAL PSYCHOLOGY
In 10 Volumes

THE NEURAL BASIS OF
THOUGHT

GEORGE G CAMPION AND
SIR GRAFTON ELLIOT SMITH

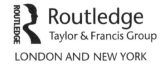

Routledge
Taylor & Francis Group

LONDON AND NEW YORK

First published in 1934
by Routledge, Trench, Trubner & Co., Ltd.
2 Park Square, Milton Park, Abingdon, Oxfordshire OX14 4RN
711 Third Avenue, New York, NY 10017

First issued in paperback 2014

Routledge is an imprint of the Taylor and Francis Group, an informa business

British Library Cataloguing in Publication Data
A CIP catalogue record for this book
is available from the British Library

The Neural Basis of Thought
ISBN 0415-21074-7
Physiological Psychology: 10 Volumes
ISBN 0415-21131-X
The International Library of Psychology: 204 Volumes
ISBN 0415-19132-7

ISBN 13: 978-1-138-87547-0 (pbk)
ISBN 13: 978-0-415-21074-4 (hbk)

ACKNOWLEDGMENTS

ACKNOWLEDGMENT is here made of permission to quote, or reproduce, from the Journals and books mentioned below, and to the Governors of the Royal Institution for the use of Sir Grafton Elliot Smith's Discourse on " The Evolution of the Mind."

The Editor of *The Journal of Philosophic Studies* (now *Philosophy*).

The Editor of *The British Journal of Psychology* (General Section).

The Editor of *The British Journal of Psychology* (Medical Section).

The Editor of *Nature*.

Miss Constance Holme, *The Lonely Plough*.

Messrs Macmillan, Wm. James' *Textbook of Psychology*.

Messrs Longmans, Green & Co., Wm. James' *Problems of Philosophy*.

Messrs Henry Holt & Co., *Principles of Psychology*.

CONTENTS

The Neural Basis of Thought

PROLOGUE

THE papers contained in this book may, from the point of view of empiricism, be regarded as an attempt to advance another step along the path of the Peirce-James-Bergson tradition. It aims at presenting the neurological aspect of a theory of knowledge which was published eleven years ago under the title *Elements in Thought and Emotion.*

These two books when read together will be found to state a theory of knowledge congruous with the ascertained mode of functioning of the various parts of the nervous system. This volume is concerned most intimately with the neurological aspect of the problem; and with the publication of Sir Grafton Elliot Smith's brilliant essay on "The Evolution of the Mind" we seem to reach a point where it may be possible to frame a fundamental psychological law or theory such as that to which William James looked forward in the final chapter of his *Textbook*—a law or theory which will lead ultimately to a unification of views which are at present conflicting, and which will embrace our cognitive and affective states of consciousness in

A   1

relation to the neural states by which they are conditioned. The chapter by Sir Grafton Elliot Smith deals with the early and continued growth processes of what is perhaps the most intricate and complex biological structure on the planet. The whole study derives mostly in the first place from William James, and later from the work and conclusions of Sir Henry Head. It began about forty years ago in an attempt to find, and after failure here, in an attempt to construct, an adequate definition of the term 'Education'—a definition which should be at once brief and comprehensive, and yet sufficiently definite and concrete to be a really practical guide to every teacher. The conclusions in which after many years these efforts issued were at length summarized in a single sentence, which in its final form ran as follows:

Education is

the Development and Discipline of

1. the body $\begin{cases} a. \text{ towards health :} \\ b. \text{ towards habits (subconscious activities)} \end{cases}$

2. the Mind with its faculties of $\left\{ \begin{array}{l} \text{acquiring,} \\ \text{differentiating,} \\ \text{correlating and} \\ \text{integrating} \end{array} \right\}$ $\left\{ \begin{array}{l} \text{percepts and} \\ \text{concepts} \end{array} \right\}$

3. the Spirit with its $\left\{ \begin{array}{l} \text{desire} \\ \text{and} \\ \text{power} \end{array} \right\}$ to use these faculties $\left\{ \begin{array}{l} \text{efficiently} \\ \text{and} \\ \text{rightly} \end{array} \right\}$

and apply them in $\left\{ \begin{array}{l} \text{controlling} \\ \text{and} \\ \text{directing} \end{array} \right\}$ the $\left\{ \begin{array}{l} \text{impulses} \\ \text{and} \\ \text{actions.} \end{array} \right\}$

This was constructed under the writer's belief that a formula could be contrived which could be shown to include all the educational influences exercised by such institutions as, the home, Pestalozzi's, Froebel's and the Montessori schools; the Scout and Guides movements; the Public schools and Universities as well as other and subsequent life and experience.

It then became necessary to work out in an essay all the implications of the above definition. This was partially done and the preliminary essay printed for private circulation in 1914, under a title suggested by an utterance of Sir Michael Sadler which appeared in the *Times Educational Supplement* for the 2nd December, 1913. "If Education," he said, "is the clue to the future it is also the Riddle of the Sphinx." The preliminary Essay was printed under the title of "The Riddle of the Sphinx." After the War it was amplified and published under the title *Elements in Thought and Emotion* (1923).

After the definition was completed and before the preliminary Essay was printed the writer became acquainted with William James' posthumous volume, published in 1911, *Some Problems in Philosophy*. In a prefatory note to this work it is stated that "two typewritten copies of this book were found after his death in August, 1910. In a memorandum dated 26th July, 1910, in which he directed the publication of the manuscript, he wrote: "Say it is fragmentary and unrevised!" "Call it 'A beginning of an introduction to philosophy.' Say that I hoped by it to round out my system, which is now too much like an arch built only on one side."

The perusal of this book and the comparing of it with his *Textbook* provided an important clue to his divergent views of the problems of knowledge with which psychology is concerned.

It would take much space to investigate this point fully, but one or two salient features of his (changed) attitude may usefully be noted.

In the Preface to his *Principles of Psychology* (1890) James had delimited the scope of the subject as he understood and expounded it. " Psychology, the science of finite individual minds, assumes as its data (1) *thoughts and feelings,* and (2) *a physical world* in time and space with which they co-exist, and which (3) *they know.*" In this larger book and the later *Textbook* he had been concerned mainly with " states of consciousness " as the subject matter of psychology, and in the final chapter of the *Textbook* (1892) in summing up the situation as he then saw it he says:

"It is strange indeed to hear people talk triumphantly of 'The New Psychology,' when into the real elements and forces which the word covers not the first glimpse of clear insight exists. A string of raw facts; a little gossip and wrangle about opinions: a little classification and generalization on the mere descriptive level: a strong prejudice that we *have* states of mind and that our brain conditions them: but not a single law in the sense in which physics shows us laws, not a single proposition from which any consequence can causally be deduced. We don't even know the terms between which the elementary laws would obtain if we had them. This is no science, it is only the hope of a science. The matter of a science is with us. Something definite happens when to a certain brain-state a certain ' sciousness ' corresponds. A genuine glimpse into what it is would be *the* scientific achievement, before which all past achievements would pale. But at present psychology is in the conditions of Physics before Galileo and the laws of motion, of chemistry and the notion that mass is preserved in all reactions. The Galileo and the Lavoisier of psychology will be famous men when indeed they come, as come they some day surely will, or past successes are no index to the future. When they do come, however, the necessities of the case will make them ' metaphysical.' Meanwhile the best way in which we can facilitate their advent is to understand how great is the darkness in which we grope, and never forget that the natural science assumptions with which we started are provisional and revisable things." [1]

In this last chapter of his *Textbook* he discusses also the relation of ' states of mind ' to ' brain states ' under the heading " Relation of Consciousness to the Brain."

" When psychology is treated as a natural science ' states of mind ' are taken for granted, as data immediately given in experience; and the working hypothesis is the mere empirical law that to the entire state of the brain at any one moment one unique state of mind always ' corresponds.' . . .

But the difficulty with the problem of ' correspondence ' is

[1] *Textbook*, 1892, p. 468.

not only that of solving it, it is that of even stating it in elementary terms. Before we can know just what sort of goings-on occur when thought corresponds to a change in the brain, we must know the *subjects* of the goings-on. We must know which sort of mental fact and which sort of cerebral fact are, so to speak, in immediate juxtaposition. We must find the minimal mental fact whose being reposes directly on a brain fact; and we must similarly find the minimal brain-event which can have a mental counterpart at all. Between the mental and physical minima thus found there will be an immediate relation, the expression of which, if we had it, would be the elementary psycho-physic law.

Our own formula has escaped the metempiric assumption of psychic atoms by *taking the entire thought* (even of a complex object) *as the minimum with which it deals on the mental side*, and the entire brain as the minimum on the physical side. But the 'entire brain' is not a physical fact at all! It is nothing but our name for the way in which a billion of molecules arranged in certain positions may affect our sense. On the principles of the corpuscular or mechanical philosophy, the only realities are the separate molecules or at most the cells. Their aggregation into a 'brain' is a fiction of popular speech. Such a figment cannot serve as the objectively real counterpart of any psychic state whatever. Only a genuinely physical fact can so serve, and the molecular fact is the only genuine physical fact. Whereupon we seem, if we are to have an elementary psycho-physic law at all, thrust right back upon something like the mental-atom-theory, for the molecular fact, being an element of the 'brain' would seem naturally to correspond, not to total thoughts, but to elements of thoughts. Thus the real in psychics seems to 'correspond' to the unreal in physics, and *vice versa*: and our perplexity is extreme."[1]

It is specially interesting to compare what he says on Conception in the *Principles* (1890) and *Textbook* (1892) with the chapters on Percept and

[1] *Textbook*, 1892, p. 464.

Concept in the *Problems of Philosophy* (1911). In The Principles we find "amid the flux of opinions and of physical things, the world of conceptions, or things intended to be thought about, stands stiff and immutable, like Plato's Realm of Ideas." (*Principles*, 1890, vol. i, p. 462.) This identical phrase is repeated word for word in the *Textbook* (1892, p. 240), but after a brief comment on what he calls " the great quarrel between nominalists and conceptualists " he ends—" In sum therefore the traditional Universal-Worship can only be called a bit of perverse sentimentalism, a philosophic ' idol of the cave ' " (p. 243). In the *Problems* (1911) no less than three chapters occupying one fourth of the book, are devoted to the subject matter " Percept and Concept." The ' Conception ' and ' Consciousness ' of the earlier books have, in these chapters written twenty years later, given place to an attempt to find and express consciousness in the reactions, interactions and mutual relationships of ' Percepts and Concepts.' His difficulties in this arise mostly from the persistent tenure in his mind of the Philosophic tradition alluded to in the phrase quoted above.

" From Aristotle downwards philosophers have frankly admitted the indispensability, for complete knowledge of fact, of both the sensational and the intellectual contribution. For complete knowledge of fact, I say, but facts are particulars and connect themselves with practical necessities and the arts; and the Greek philosophers soon formed the notion that a knowledge of so-called ' universals ' consisting of concepts of abstract forms, qualities, numbers, and relations was the only knowledge worthy of the truly philosophic mind. Particular facts decay and our perceptions of them vary. A concept never varies; and between such unvarying terms the relations must be constant and express eternal verities. Hence there arose a tendency, which has lasted all through philosophy, to contrast the knowledge of universals and intelligibles, as god-like, dignified, and honourable to the knower, with that of particulars and sensibles as something relatively base which more or less allies us with the beasts. . . .

. . . For rationalistic writers conceptual knowledge was not only the more noble knowledge, but it originated independently of all perceptual particulars. Such concepts as God, perfection, eternity, infinity, immutability, identity, absolute beauty, truth, justice, necessity, freedom, duty, worth, etc., and the part they play in our mind, are, it was supposed, impossible to explain as results of practical experience. The empiricist view, and probably the true view, is that they do result from practical experience."[1]

James in this later book continues to use the term ' concept ' in the sense of the Platonic ' Universal '; a static rigid mental entity which never varies; yet in discussing the relations and interactions of percepts and concepts his analogies sometimes bring him nearly to the view of organic growth: *e.g.* (p. 80) " Whether our concepts live by returning to the perceptual world or not, they live by having come from it. It is the nourishing ground from which their sap is drawn." Side by side and in contrast with these should

[1] *Problems of Philosophy*, pp. 54-5.

be placed his remark after quoting with approval Steinthal's account of changes in the 'apperceiving mass' of Herbart—changes produced by the assimilation of new data acquired in perception. "This account of Steinthal's brings out very clearly the *difference between our psychological Conceptions and what are called concepts in logic.* In logic a concept is unalterable, but what are popularly called our 'conceptions of things' alter by being used. The aim of 'Science' is to attain conceptions so adequate and exact that we shall never need to change them. There is an everlasting struggle in every mind between the tendency to keep unchanged and the tendency to renovate our ideas. Our education is a ceaseless compromise between the conservative and the progressive factors."[1]

Dr F. C. S. Schiller in his various criticisms of formal logic has given expression to the feeling that the growth of psychological and biological knowledge must profoundly transform traditional epistemology, and the studies herein contained are offered as a contribution to this end.

In the view here presented the concept is for long periods of the individual life continually changing by a process of organic growth. It is also ineradicably subjective and the means by which we construct alike our statements of what

[1] *Textbook*, p. 327.

on the one hand we call ' fact ' and on another
hand we call ' fancy.' In the process of perception the growth takes place by the active selection
of relevant data from the passing perceptual
pageant as a monkey seizes nuts from their surroundings in jumping from tree to tree. An
illustration of this process in the individual mind
is presented in Chapter III. A little reflection
will easily convince us that if this is true in the
mind of the individual a similar process is also at
work in the collective mind of the race. The
Ptolemaic conception of the Universe gave way
to the Copernican. The Newtonian system of
Nature has in the course of a hundred years
broken down under the stress of new observations
accumulating into a growing body of thought
inconsistent with the premises from which the
newer observations were made.

The concepts which, in their several and individual processes of growth and in their ever-
changing relations to one another, collectively go
to make up our varying processes of thought,
provide by their very subjectivity the means of
explaining the whole universe of human error,
human illusion, and human self-deception. Any
theory of experience which fails in this is fore-
doomed to failure as an attempt to explain what
is commonly regarded as human knowledge.
These discrete elements of thought grow into our

minds in childhood and outgrow later the illusions which they engender. These illusions must be regarded as necessary and therefore excellent stages in the growth from mental childhood to mental maturity. All will agree that the problem of the genesis and growth of human knowledge is quite a different one from that of the nature and validity of human truth. In the writer's view the theory to which he has gradually attained is at best only a statement of the errorful subjectivity of human knowledge and of the doubtful probability of an adequate philosophic theory of Truth being ever reached in terms of that knowledge. Of the trans-subjective inferences which must enter into any complete theory of epistemology an admirable sketch will be found in the recently published Balfour Lectures on Realism (3rd series) by the late Prof. A. Seth Pringle Pattison.

William James gave it as a ' general law ' of perception that " *whilst part of what we perceive comes through our senses from the object before us, another part* (and it may be the larger part) *always comes out of our own mind.*" [1] But this general law is entirely lacking in the refinement necessary to express the gradation observable in the varying amount of the conceptual contribution in any given act of perception. It is more adequately

[1] *Textbook,* p. 329.

stated in a paragraph (p. 38) from the chapter on Sense-Perception in my book *Elements in Thought and Emotion*:

" There is great truth, but not the whole truth, in the old saying that a man sees in any view or picture or other work of art what his mind brings to the examination of it. A sculptor in the galleries of the British Museum will see in the Elgin Marbles the beauty of form and line which mark them as precious fragments of the creative genius of one of the great art periods of human history. A child among the same statues may see only at the same moment ' a glorious place to play hide and seek.' And the complementary truth is that the growth from one condition to the other is brought about by the gradual refinement of the power of differential perception of the visual sense-data with the aid of the ever-extending and more highly-differentiated conceptual contents of the mind."

The thesis of this book is that the multitudinous and diverse concepts in their equally multitudinous and diverse groupings have their neural counterparts in what Sir Henry Head has called ' neural schemata.' These neural schemata are patterns of neural impulse, not indeed such as can be dissected out and displayed anatomically like the blood-vessels, but inferred and functional entities resembling in this respect the biological ' genes.' A neural schema has in the course of an individual lifetime been formed for each concept which the mind acquires; these multitudinous schemata are severally connected (1) peripherally with one or more of our receptor sense organs, and (2) centrally with the thalami and other basal ganglia; so that a nervous impulse passing through these schemata, whether from the receptor sense organs or from the thalami, brings into what we call consciousness [1] the particular concept or series of concepts which have become in the course of the individual life associated with the neural schemata being so activated. The continuity and diversity of what we call our thought-processes is secured by the alternating circulation of neural impulse through these multitudinous neural schemata from the thalami and other basal ganglia to the cortex and then back to the thalami by the cortico-thalamic paths. The detailed nature of this among other circulations of neural impulse in the brain are explained more fully in Sir Grafton Elliot Smith's chapter on "The Evolution of the Mind."

[1] Exceptions to this are numerous especially in psycho-pathic cases.

CHAPTER I

THE EVOLUTION OF THE MIND [1]

BY SIR GRAFTON ELLIOT SMITH F.R.S.

IT may be asked by what right an anatomist, whose proper business is concerned with very concrete subjects, presumes to discuss so elusive and immaterial a subject as the evolution of the mind, even if it be admitted that the evolution of the chief organ of the mind comes within the proper scope of his field of work. I am encouraged, however, to embark on this hazardous attempt by the considered judgment of Prof. S. Alexander, who once expressed the opinion " that we are forced to go beyond the mere correlation of the mental with [the] neural processes and to identify them."

The great physiologist who is most competent to express an opinion on this issue has recently impressed upon us the need for caution in touching it. In the closing passage of his Rede Lecture

[1] This chapter was delivered as a Friday Evening Discourse at the Royal Institution on January 19, 1934, and was published in Volume XXVIII of the Proceedings of the Royal Institution and as a special supplement of *Nature* on February 17, 1934. I am indebted to the Royal Institution and the Editor of *Nature* for permission to reprint the Discourse here.

on " The Brain and Its Mechanism," delivered in Cambridge on December 5, 1933, Sir Charles Sherrington used these words: " I reflect with apprehension that a great subject can revenge itself shrewdly for being too hastily touched. To the question of the relation between brain and mind the answer given by a physiologist sixty years ago was ' ignorabimus.' But to-day less than yesterday do we think the definite limits of exploration yet attained. The problem I have so grossly touched has one virtue at least, it will long offer to those who pursue it the comfort that to journey is better than to arrive, but that comfort assumes arrival. Some of us—perhaps because we are too old—or is it too young?—think there may be arrival at last." These opinions are even more appropriate to those who lack Sir Charles Sherrington's immense competence.

Hence I seize upon a confession made by Sir Charles elsewhere in his Rede Lecture:

" What right have we to conjoin mental experience with physiological? No scientific right; only the right of what Keats, with that superlative Shakespearian gift of his, dubbed ' busy common sense.' The right which practical life, naïve and shrewd, often exercises."

If scientific proof, however, is demanded, surely Sir Henry Head's investigation of sensation and the cerebral cortex supplies it by demonstrating in wounded soldiers the concern of the cortex with psychical functions—the dependence of mind on brain (*Studies in Neurology*, 1920). Prof. Shaw Bolton, by comparative and clinico-pathological researches, has demonstrated the dependence of mind on the supragranular layer of the cerebral cortex.

With these assurances the mere biologist, while discussing strictly biological issues, can direct attention to certain psychological implications of anatomical facts and comment also on their neurological aspects for the interpretation of the mind and its working. In previous lectures at the Royal Institution I have discussed the significance of the heightened powers of vision in man's ancestors, which conferred upon them the ability to see the world in which they were living and appreciate something of what was happening in it, as well as to guide their hands to acquire skill, by the practice of which fresh knowledge and understanding were obtained.

Significance of Visual Guidance

We know enough of the comparative anatomy and palæontology of the Primates to select a series of animals that can be taken to represent approximately the stages through which man's ancestors passed in their evolution towards man's estate, and by examining the connexions of the optic tracts in the brain, arrive at an understanding of what is involved in the acquisition of higher powers of visual discrimination (Fig. 1).

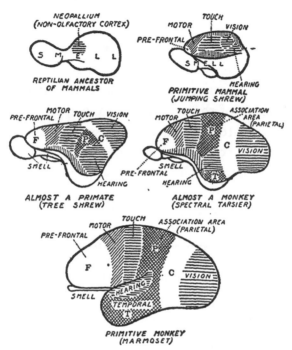

FIG. 1.—A series of diagrams to suggest the origin of the neopallium in the ancestor of mammals; the rapid development of this cortical area in mammals, as touch, vision, hearing, as well as control of skilled movements, attain an increasing significance, the growing cultivation of vision which leads to the emergence of the Primates, the increased reliance on vision brings about an enhancement of skill in movement (and a marked expansion of the motor territory) and of tactile and auditory discrimination. (Based in part on the work of Profs. W. E. Le Gros Clark and H. H. Woollard.) From *Human History* (1930).

In this series of diagrams, it will be observed that at first the areas for touch, vision and hearing

B

come into contact with one another but that eventually an area marked P (parietal association area) develops between them to provide a more efficient place of blending of the impulses from these three senses. At the same time there emerges from the front end of the brain a prefrontal area (F) which is essentially an outgrowth of the motor territory and an instrument whereby the activities of the whole cortex can in some way be concentrated on the process of learning to give motor expression to the total activities of the hemisphere. Certain poisons which exert a destructive influence on the supragranular layer of this part of the cortex lead to very significant mental results, such as are displayed in general paralysis of the insane, characterized at first by grandiose delusions and afterwards by a failure of the mental process altogether, profound dementia. The discussion of this evidence by Dr J. Shaw Bolton (*The Brain in Health and Disease*, 1914) affords another precise demonstration of the dependence of the mind upon particular parts of the brain.

This is an example of the means whereby comparative anatomy can throw light upon the process of mental evolution, the structural changes in the eyes and brain which make possible not only the refinement of visual discrimination, but also the increasing participation of visual percep-

tion in the conscious life and in the guidance of
the instruments (such as the hands) of muscular
skill. The latter consideration is one of fundamental importance. For the study of the evolution of the nervous system impresses upon us the
fact that one of its essential purposes is to make
possible quicker, more complex and more pur-
posive responses to changes in the animal's environment or the conditions in its own body.

It is a matter of real importance, therefore, that
every advance in the powers of sensory perception
and discrimination should be brought into relationship with this essential biological need of
finding expression in action. Each of the major
advances in vertebrate evolution is obviously
correlated with differences in locomotion and
muscular aptitude. When an amphibian emerged
from a fish-like ancestor, the most obtrusive
change was the substitution for swimming as a
means of locomotion, the use of the newly-created
' gadgets ' which are represented by the limbs of
a tetrapod land-living animal. The attainment
of greater competence and agility in the control
of the amphibian's four legs led to the emergence
of reptiles, from which in course of time birds and
mammals were evolved; the former by high
specialization of the forelimbs by flight, and the
latter by the acquisition of a cerebral instrument,
the neopallium, which conferred the ability to

attain unlimited powers of acquiring skill and to profit from experience. The highest powers of skill were made possible by the evolution of greater powers of visual guidance.

It is an obvious truism that man's mental superiority is largely the outcome of the perfection of the co-operation of hand and eye in the attainment of manipulative skill and dexterity. In the use of the hands for the expression of skill, the skin of the fingers acquires heightened powers of tactile discrimination, and thus becomes the special organ of the sense of touch and an instrument of perceptual knowledge second only to the eyes in significance.

The researches of Sir Henry Head and his collaborators have given us a new understanding of what is involved in tactile discrimination. The great sensory pathways in the spinal cord and brain-stem lead up to the thalamus in the forebrain, where they end in its ventral nucleus, the nerve cells of which transmit impulses in two directions—one to the cerebral cortex and the other to what Sir Henry Head calls the essential organ of the thalamus. The former is regarded by him as the mechanism for sensory discrimination, and the latter as the instrument for awareness to sensation and the appreciation of its affective qualities, its pleasantness or unpleasantness.

Hypothesis of a Thalamo-Cortical Circulation

In the *British Journal of Medical Psychology* in 1929, Mr George G. Campion discussed the psychological implications of Head's clinical results. Emphasizing the impossibility of separating from perception the affective factor, which is continually at work in our thought-processes, Mr Campion gave expression to the view that the biological purpose of giving a meaning to experience is the essence of the comprehension of the nature of sensation. Mr Campion has emphasized the further fact that the concept—the ultimate constituent element of what are called our cognitive dispositions—is not fixed and unchangeable, but is " a living plastic mental symbol subject to a process of organic growth, and that its growth is due to an affective factor which is constantly at work determining the selection of new sense data from the perpetual flux, interpenetrating the conceptual contents of our minds, and integrating all these various and varying constituents into the slowly maturing dispositions which constitute organized knowledge. The affective factor involved in this process has been variously called ' libido,' ' love,' ' interest,' ' feeling,' ' desire,' ' liking,' etc."

Mr Campion further maintains that there is a

continuous stream of neural impulses from the thalamus to the cortex and from the cortex to the thalamus, which keeps alive this living process of mental growth—the enrichment of the concept as the result of personal experience, the success or failure of the attempts to do things.

Developing this idea, Mr Campion directs attention to the various parts of the cortex linked in an incredibly complicated way by association fibres and cortical association areas. The necessary implication of his hypothesis of the thalamo-cortical circulation of neural impulses (by means of the various thalamo-cortical and cortico-thalamic tracts of fibres), involves functional connexions of the various parts of the thalamus with one another by intercommunicating fibres. He predicts that as " the cortical association areas may be assumed to have a counterpart also in the thalami, it will be for neurologists to say whether these hypothetical association areas lie in and constitute a chief part of what Head has called the essential thalamic organs."

Since this prediction was made, Prof. Le Gros Clark, in the course of studies (*Brain*, vol. 55) in the comparative anatomy and physiology of the thalamus, has directed attention to the fact that such elements are actually found in the thalamus of the higher mammalia. There are cell masses (lateral nucleus (Fig. 3)) deriving their impulses from the main sensory part (ventral nucleus) of the thalamus, which merge sensory impulses of different kinds and establish direct connexions with those association areas of the cortex which link together the cortical sensory areas. This remarkable confirmation of Mr Campion's hypothesis adds force to the argument that the mechanism of correlation in the thalamus is far more complicated than has hitherto been supposed, and represents what, following the lead of Sir Henry Head, one may suppose to be a mechanism for the integration of affective processes in the same way as the cortex effects the integration of the discriminative or cognitive aspects of experience.

In the process of acquiring knowledge and building up these vital mental elements, the concepts, to which reference has already been made, it is obvious that there must be a circulation of nervous impulses such as Mr Campion assumes to maintain the cohesion and the integrity of the vital processes of thought. This circulation of impulses must be even more complicated than he has assumed, because the hypothalamus undoubtedly enters into the process and influences the activities both of the thalamus and the cortex, adding as its quota the visceral element which confers upon experience an emotional factor which is something more than the affective interest the

thalamus is able to provide. Intimately inter-
twined with the whole of this complicated system
—hypothalamus, thalamus and the sensory and
association areas of the cortex—we have the
complex mechanism for giving expression to their
combined activities in actions which represent the
biological purpose of the whole process. The
powerful instrument of thought represented by
speech affords an admirable illustration of the
intimate correlation of muscular skill with cognitive
aptitude to provide the essential currency of mind.

Almost every part of the cerebral cortex is
intimately connected directly and indirectly with
mechanisms in the central nervous system which
are concerned with muscular activities, either those
which directly effect movements, or on a vastly
greater scale those which prepare and co-ordinate
the state of the muscles of the whole body in
readiness for prompt and efficient action. More
than two-thirds of the fibres that leave the hemisphere have as their immediate purpose the
establishment of connexions with the cerebellum,
and as their function, the rapid distribution of
the muscular tone of the body in readiness for
such skilled action as lies at the root of the brain's
efficiency. The circulation of the thalamic and
cortical currents maintains this constant state of
readiness and is a vital and essential part of consciousness and mind.

The building up in the brain of concepts is dependent not merely on affective and cognitive experience based upon afferent impulses from the sense organs, but is also brought about as the result of muscular activity, the doing things with the hands, the gradual perfecting of the movements, the results of the success or failure of such efforts, and the afferent impulses which pour into the brain from the joints, the muscles and the skin areas to record the success or failure of particular muscular activities. It is largely by doing things that experience is built up. It is important therefore to recognize the very large part which such conative activities play in the building up of concepts. They are due not merely to the interaction of the affective and cognitive dispositions, but also to the dynamic factor which is conferred upon these processes by attempting to express in action the result of the discriminative activities of the cortex.

The Neopallium as the Essential Mental Instrument

More than thirty years ago, I directed attention to the fact (*J. Anat. and Physiol.*, p. 431; 1901) that with the evolution of mammals a new cortical instrument, which I called the neopallium, came into existence, and with its expansion provoked the vastest revolution that ever occurred in the cerebral structure. It came into being to form a receptive organ for fibres coming from the thalamus, whereby touch, vision, hearing and taste— in fact all the non-olfactory senses—secured representation in the cerebral cortex. To express this fact, Prof. Winkler, of Utrecht, calls the neopallium the thalamocortex.

In its earliest form the neopallium consists of a tiny area far forward in the hemisphere, where tactile impulses from the lips and tongue are brought into relationship with olfactory and gustatory impulses, and this area afterwards acquires the ability to control the movements of the lips and tongue. As the neopallium grows it establishes similar relations to the rest of the body and increases the range of its receptive powers not merely to the skin of the whole body, but also to the eyes and ears, and it establishes direct connexions with all the motor nuclei in the central nervous system. The neopallium not only gives the senses other than smell representation in the dominant part of the brain, and a part in the control of behaviour, but it also provides a continuous territory in which co-operation between these various sensory influences can be established and their conjoint effects be brought to bear upon the mechanisms that control motor activities.

It is often supposed that there are in the cerebral

cortex long association bundles to establish connexions between distant parts of the cerebral
cortex. There has recently been published an
important memoir by Dr Stephen Poljak, a Yugo-
slav neurologist who began the research in question
in my laboratory eight years ago, which disproves
the existence of such long connexions. An impulse
from one cortical area can only reach and influence
distant areas by travelling through the cortex
itself. The act of correlation involves the
whole cortex. Even in the simplest act of thought
or skill, the whole neopallium participates. The
manifold currents which circulate throughout
the brain in the process of regulating muscular
activities represent the means of integrating the
cognitive, affective and conative activities in
thought.

Not only the neopallium but also the brain as
a whole adds its quota to the action—in particular
the great mass of nervous matter at the threshold
of the cerebral hemisphere known as the thalamus.
It contributes the affective element, which is the
interest, the stimulative of the whole complex
process, to which it gives coherence. The cortex
not only preserves the records of previous experience which provide the means for comparing
present experiences with past happenings, but it
also adds the spatial quality to sensation and the
means of judging degrees of stimulation, and the

afferent impulses which pour into the brain from the joints, the muscles and the skin areas, to record the success or failure of particular muscular activities. It is by doing things that experience is built up. It is important therefore to recognize the very large part which such conative activities play in the building up of concepts. They are due not merely to the interaction of the affective and cognitive dispositions, but also to the dynamic factor which is conferred upon these processes by attempting to express in action the result of the discriminative activities of the cortex.

For some years I have been attempting to demonstrate how vast a part the cultivation of visual discrimination has played, not simply in making it possible for human beings to see the world in which they live and appreciate some of the activities which are revealed to them by their eyes, but even more in contributing to conscious control of behaviour.

The earliest type of cerebral cortex necessarily has to perform both affective and cognitive functions. It enables its possessor to appreciate the attractiveness or unattractiveness of a particular scent, and to experience an interest in addition to the cognitive recognition of it.

The cortex, at first, however, exercises no immediate direction over the motor activities of the animal beyond provoking them and providing the initiative to action. This it accomplishes by transmitting to a mass of grey matter in its base (the corpus striatum) impulses which indirectly throw other parts of the brain and spinal cord into action to direct the movements that it starts. It is the impulses from the eyes, skin and ' ears ' (as yet organs not of hearing, but of recording movements in the water) which consciously direct

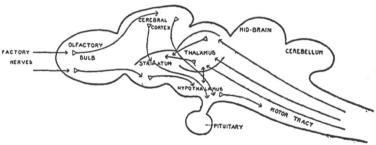

FIG. 2.—Diagram of the primitive vertebrate brain to suggest the hypothalamic, thalamic, striatal and cortical connexions.

the animal's movements, while its posture and equilibrium are being maintained by the automatic mechanism of the membranous labyrinth.

The tracts in the brain which convey the impulses from skin, eyes and ears are mainly concerned with transmitting to the various motor nuclei impulses that unconsciously influence and direct reflex movements, but they all send some of their impulses to a mass of grey matter in the forebrain, which lies immediately behind the striatum, to which it is intimately linked by many nerve fibres. This is the thalamus (Fig. 2). It confers upon all the non-olfactory sensory impulses an affective quality which gives them a meaning and an influence in modifying behaviour. In other words, the effects of this sensory experience, when transmitted to the striatum, are to alter the animal's reactions to smell.

Emotional Factor in Mind

The activities of the striatum, when stimulated by the cerebral hemispheres and the thalamus, are expressed in impulses which proceed from it to the hypothalamus, a mass of grey matter lying beneath the thalamus. This surprising arrangement seems to confer upon the hypothalamus the decisive influence in translating into behaviour the initiative to action which lies in the cerebral cortex. The hypothalamus is the part of the brain which controls, by means of the sympathetic and parasympathetic systems, the most vital activities of the body itself, its visceral functions, its growth and metabolism, and even such appetites as those of sex. It is the essential instrument of emotional expression.

As the springs of action are profoundly influenced by hunger, thirst, sexual desire and other appetites and cravings, it is perhaps not surprising that in the most primitive vertebrates the instrument of the animal's vegetative needs should play a crucial part in shaping its conduct. To this part of the brain, impulses proceed from the olfactory tracts so as directly to control the activities of the alimentary and genital systems in anticipation of the realization of the satisfaction of the respective appetites.

The study of the primitive brain impresses upon us the intimacy of the integration of the functions concerned with affective and discriminative knowledge and the translation of such information into appropriate action.

The higher type of brain distinctive of mammals, which opens up the possibility of the attainment of real conceptual knowledge and its biological application in increasingly complex acts of skill and thought, is distinguished by the growth of the thalamus and the transmission from it to the cerebral cortex of fibres in increasing numbers (Fig. 3).

The recent progress in our knowledge of the structure and connexions of the thalamus and hypothalamus with the cerebral cortex, the hypothalamus and the sympathetic and visceral tracts of the organism had made it possible to carry Mr Campion's suggestions a stage further than he himself has done. That this is possible is in large measure due to the illuminating researches of Prof. W. E. Le Gros Clark. The intensive studies which have recently been made by scores of investigators on the structure and connexions of the hypothalamus enable us to broaden the issues and consider the part played by these portions of the brain, which control the growth and meta-

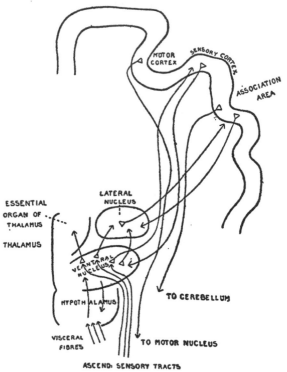

FIG. 3.—Diagram of the thalamic, hypothalamic and cortical connexions of the human brain.

bolism of the body, and in particular visceral function, and how they are related to the thalamus and the cerebral cortex and provide the instrument for determining the emotional colour of experience and of regulating the manifestations of the appetites.

If Mr Campion's views are correct, that the study of this neural machinery is essential for the understanding and interpretation of thought and behaviour, its structure and functions might be expected to be of great complexity. Hence it becomes essential to look at the whole issue from a much broader point of view than the mere connexions of thalamus and cerebral cortex.

IMPORTANCE OF SMELL IN THE PRIMITIVE VERTEBRATE

In the brain of the most primitive vertebrate, the structural pattern is determined by the fact that smell is the dominant sense. The cerebral cortex is essentially a receptive instrument for impressions of smell, and the mechanism whereby consciousness of smell can influence the behaviour of the animal. When a primitive vertebrate such as a dogfish scents attractive food and pursues it, the culmination of the pursuit is represented by the seizure of the food and the appreciation of its taste. This is nearly akin to the initial olfactory experience which started the pursuit and dominated it, so that all the incidents of the pursuit become integrated into one experience, which is thus given coherence and meaning. Thus is initiated the ability to anticipate the result of a given course of action, and to recall in memory the connexion between the various incidents.

c

One must assume, therefore, that the primitive cortex is concerned not merely with the awareness of smell and the ability to discriminate between different kinds of smells, but also that it is concerned with the affective side of olfactory experience, with the attractiveness or repulsiveness of any scent and the influence of such affective experience in determining the nature of the response an individual odour can evoke. The cerebral cortex in such a primitive animal is incapable of directing movements, seeing that the sense of smell is utterly devoid of any spatial quality. When an animal scents an attractive food, it acquires from the sense of smell no idea as to the position in space of the object which provides the stimulus. It is merely stirred into action, and other neural mechanisms are responsible for controlling and directing the resulting activities. The cerebral cortex, so to speak, is the mere trigger which releases the activity of the brain and provokes and directs the movements.

The part of the cerebral hemisphere which translates these stimuli into action is the corpus striatum, and the striatum is connected with the thalamus, which receives from the body, that is through the skin, the eyes and the ears as well as the muscles and joints, impulses which modify and direct movements that result when the animal is thrown into action. The thalamus transmits the effects of these stimuli to the striatum and so modifies the motor activities. In the case of organs such as the eyes, the primary functions were concerned not merely with the awareness of illumination, but also of movements in the outside world, or rather movements of objects in the outside world in reference in its own body. The eyes have associated with them, in the brain, a complicated mechanism which enables them automatically to direct the movements of the body in relationship to events in the outside world. But quite apart from this, the eyes transmit to a part of the thalamus (the lateral geniculate body) impulses which are concerned with the awareness of the stimulus of light, and which influence these bodies and through them the thalamus as a whole, which in turn affects the functions of the striatum and the movements of the animal.

In the primitive vertebrate one must assume that the thalamus acts as an affective organ of all senses other than smell, and represents the instrument whereby the organism is pleasantly or unpleasantly affected by sensory experience, and that the cerebral cortex performs the analogous but more dominating aspect of the same function in relationship with smell. The dominant part of the cerebral cortex in the most primitive vertebrate is the hippocampal formation, and if one assumes the supreme function of the cortex is to determine the behaviour of the animal, it is perhaps justifiable to assume that the purpose of the primitive hippocampus is to make possible the adequate association of the affective qualities of smell and to translate them into action by playing a dominant part in determining the animal's behaviour.

It is perhaps not without significance in this connexion that the efferent fibres from the hippocampal formation, after passing out of the cerebral hemisphere, terminate in the hypothalamus, that part of the brain which controls the visceral system (sympathetic and para-sympathetic) and thereby regulates the activity of the viscera. It is, in fact, that part of the brain which is intimately related to the functions of the appetites. Nor is it surprising that the particular part of the hypothalamus in which the hippocampal fibres terminate should be linked up with the thalamus, so as to provide a neural circuit in which the total affective qualities of all the senses are brought into relationship in such a way that they can influence through the striatum the motor responses of the body.

The researches of Prof. Le Gros Clark have established the fact that the thalamus contains three kinds of cell groups (Fig. 2). Those forming the ultimate termini of certain of the sensory pathways, which according to Sir Henry Head form the essential organ of the thalamus, are the instrument whereby we become aware of sensory experience and appreciate its affective qualities. Secondly, there is a group of cells (ventral nucleus) which receives the great sensory paths coming up from the other parts of the brain and the spinal cord, and transmits the impulses either to the corpus striatum or in mammals to the neopallium. In the third place, there is a group of nuclei in the thalamus which become well developed only in the higher mammals. They do not receive afferent impulses directly, but only from the intermediation of the ventral nucleus. The highest type of thalamic cells, known as the lateral nucleus (Fig. 3), establishes connexions with the parietal area of the neopallium, which intervenes between the sensory cortical areas for touch, vision and hearing (*P*, Fig. 1), and presumably confers upon this area the ability to provide sensory experience with spatial and discriminative qualities. All three categories of thalamic elements are intimately joined together by numerous fibre tracts so as to form a closely integrated functional whole, the proper working of which is essential for cortical functions.

INTEGRATION OF THE DISPOSITIONS OF THE MIND

The common practice of psychologists of segregating the three dispositions of the mind, cognitive, affective and conative, and attempting to study them as isolated units, is devoid of justification. All three are indissolubly united in the working of the mind. To give them cohesion it is necessary to assume the existence of a circulation of nervous impulses from the thalamus to the cortex and to the widespread and complex mechanisms concerned with muscular activities.

In the growth of a concept conation plays a fundamental part. Man learns from experimentation. By the exercise of his manual dexterity he acquires knowledge of the properties of things, the nature of forces, and the means for interpreting (and in some measure understanding) the world in which he lives. The surprisingly large part of the cerebral cortex that is concerned with the regulation of muscular functions and the multitude of its fibre-connexions with the cerebellum affords an impressive testimony of the vast significance of action in mind-making and emphasizes what Prof. T. H. Pear has well called " the intellectual respectability of muscular skill." It is a truism that we learn by doing. In man, thought is a prerequisite for action, and action a corrective of thought. The biological justification for the evolution of the high degree of visual discrimination, whereby man knows the world and the society in which he lives, is the motor efficiency it makes possible.

The most significant factor in the evolution of the mind was effected when the direction of movements was transferred from the midbrain to the neopallium (see *Nature*, 125, p. 820; 1930) and from being an unconscious automatism became a consciously directed process. For the neopallium not only established a direct control over the motor nuclei of the whole central nervous system, but it also became linked up with all the complicated machinery in other parts of the brain which is concerned with muscular activites.

This concentration of control in the neopallium implies a circulation of nervous impulses throughout the brain to effect cohesion between the living instruments of the conative dispositions with those of the affective (thalamus) and cognitive (neopallium) dispositions of the mind. A circulation such as Mr Campion postulates is essential to the working of the mind.

This circulation in turn involves the hypothalamus, which presumably confers the emotional tone that plays a part in all mental and muscular activity, in particular in artistic expression and the self-knowledge which is one of the most distinctive qualities of man and his thinking.

Anthropological investigations, the results of which I have summarized in chaps. v and vi of my *Human History* (1930), suggest that in primitive man there is an innate goodness and truthfulness, the awareness of which we call conscience. These qualities of the mind are responsible for character and personality. The terrible experiments which the incidence of diseases such as sleepy sickness (encephalitis lethargica) provides, has shown that these amiable qualities can be destroyed by minute injuries of certain parts of the brain in or in the neighbourhood of the hypothalamus. We must suppose that these parts of the brain are responsible for the maintenance of the innate goodness of human nature, the goodwill of normal man, seeing that their destruction causes so profound an alteration of character. Mr Campion's hypothesis of a widespread circulation of nervous impulses provides an explanation of how these various dispositions of the mind and character may be integrated into the living human personality.

Before I close this discourse, I must express my gratitude to Mr George Campion for his stimulating suggestions and to Prof. J. S. B. Stopford, of Manchester, for help in giving them neurological expression.

CHAPTER II

THE term ' concept ' as used to-day in Psychology I understand to carry with it no special and exclusive reference to the Platonic ' universal.' I rather suppose it to be used in a wider sense and I adopt the view expressed by Prof. J. B. Pratt in his essay on " The Possibility of Knowledge," where he says, " How indeed can we think at all? Surely only by means of concepts! The concept is thus not the object of one's thought but the means of one's thinking, and to have a concept of one's friend *is* to think of him." [1]

Entirely congruous with this usage of Prof. Pratt is the view that ' knowledge is experience mediated by mental symbols '—symbols which we severally denote by what the logicians call ' terms.' These symbols, abstracted from experience and providing the means of acquiring further and new experience, have from time to time in the history of philosophy been introduced and reintroduced under various collective terms of which ' concept ' is only one. Call them what we will—' ideas,' ' concepts,' ' presentations,' ' repre-

[1] *Essays in Critical Realism,* p. 97.

sentations,' ' images,' ' notions '—assign to them
an utterly negligible place in any theory of truth
and they must be still regarded as our veritable
means of thinking much as racquets and balls
are means of playing tennis and different kinds
of measuring devices are means of accurate and
studied observation. As without racquets and
balls we cannot play tennis and as without measuring instruments we cannot measure, so without
concepts we cannot think.

These symbols may, moreover, be weighted
with different kinds of what we usually call
' imagery.' This imagery may be visual, auditory,
audito-motor, tactile, motile, or kinaesthetic, or
the symbols may be entirely ' abstract '; and I
believe I shall be impugning no recognized tenet
of psychology in holding the view that of such
mental symbols in multitudinous, diverse and ever-
changing clusterings and groupings our entire
cognitive dispositions are ultimately composed.

In the usage of traditional philosophy ' concepts ' as ' universals ' have been regarded as
static, stable, unchanging mental entities in an
ever-changing universe of perceptual flux. Prof.
Spearman in his book on the *Nature of Intelligence*
alludes to this traditional usage of the term and
presents it in a vivid and picturesque phrase.
" Conception," he remarks, " may be said to
possess no brush or palate but only a box of

mosaic stones," [1] and if we amplify his metaphor we may conceive of our entire cognitive dispositions as a variegated and widely extended mosaic pavement displaying a series of complicated and inextricably interwoven patterns.

Now the view to which I ask your consideration is how much more congruous with our ordinary experience it will be if we regard each and all of the stones composing this mosaic pavement *not* as static, stable units but as living mental entities subject to a process of organic growth; and to illustrate what I have in mind I take one of the concepts which go to make up my own series of cognitive dispositions, and the one which I select is that of a recent President of the British Association—Sir Arthur Keith.

My concept of him began about a quarter of a century ago as an entirely nebulous conception consisting of little more than a name and a belief that this name indicated the existence of some human personality. There was, too, a belief that this personality had been answerable for the publication of a volume on the subject of Embryology. The concept remained for some time, possibly for some few years, in this inchoate and nebulous state, and then it began a process of growth which has continued up to the present time. One day I made what we call the personal

[1] *The Nature of Intelligence and the Principles of Cognition*, p. 265.

acquaintance of this nebulous being, and my concept was enlarged and enriched by means of a large and complex series of additions which it acquired by a multitudinous series of new perceptions in a personal interview at the College of Surgeons. The concept by means of this new perceptual experience made a great spurt of growth and became endowed with entirely new qualities, visual, auditory, tactile. Its inchoate and nebulous condition became changed to a more highly differentiated complexity, or to express it in Spencerian phrase it was passing from a condition of " indefinite incoherent homogeneity to one of a definite coherent heterogeneity." The process thus begun has continued over a period of twenty years and always in essentially the same way—by a process of selective acquisition of new data available in the manifold continuum of the perceptual flux. The sources and conditions have been various. From some of his many works, from articles in the press, from letters, or from the more complex series of percepts acquired during personal intercourse. And although during its twenty or twenty-five years' growth this concept has become a highly differentiated complexity of different parts and qualities it has nevertheless retained its original and essential unity—a unity enriched and revalued from time to time as the years have passed and occupying a profoundly different position in my entire series of cognitive dispositions to that which it originally held.

A little reflection will make it apparent that in this process of growth which has been taking place in the concept there is a strange similarity to the kind of growth which takes place in the material being of all of us, a growth in mass or bulk accompanied by a wondrously differentiated complexity both of structure and of function. Nor will it seem strange that a growth-process, which has to be studied over a period reckoned in decades, may well appear non-existent in the seconds or parts of a second which are the duration of some of the experiments of the psychological laboratory.

But besides this growth-process in the concept a more subtle change has also gradually been taking place in it. It has become shot through and through with some emotional element which has been largely the cause of the growth and has besides gone far to convert it into an ' affect.' And thus the mere name which has always been attached to it, and indeed may be regarded as a part of it, suffices to direct my ' attention ' to and enchain it for the time upon the sense data in any new perceptual experience which have reference to even one of its many parts.

Now this continual action of an emotional element in causing the growth of concepts has hardly received the experimental study which is its due, and finds perhaps inadequate place in some of the traditional terms of the psychological textbooks. It is easy for a formal and mechanistic logic to draw on paper its distinction between the denotation and connotations of a term, but in life these are mingled in every act of reflection and expression. It is easy for psychology to categorize our minds into cognitive, conative and affective dispositions, but to do this is *ipso facto* to falsify them unless, while using these terms, we keep constantly in mind that their unity is more endur-ing and fundamental than this division: that these ancient mental categories may present admirable examples of the rigorous purity of philosophical abstraction but are thereby detached from the unceasing change and intermingling of their elements which unite them inextricably in the life of thought, feeling and action. No concept can pass in thought without being in some degree interfused with some emotional tinge and no conative or affective process takes place without its complement of conceptual elements. The clue to the resolution of these abstractions lies, as Prof. Spearman has said, in a comprehensive theory of cognition, and such a theory will, from the neces-sities of the case, regard the mental symbols or concepts which go to make up our cognitive dis-positions as living and growing mental entities both stimulated into activity by, and acquiring new elements of mental growth from, the sense data being continually presented in the continuum of the perceptual flux.

In the past two decades the tide of investigation and study in Psychology has swung from the course which James was pursuing at the time of his death to the new and fruitful range of discovery initiated by Freud, and its application in the sphere of psycho-pathology. This has in some ways diverted attention for the time being from the problem of the nature of cognition, but when attention becomes again focused on this problem Freud's work will assuredly be found to have assisted in breaking down the sterile abstractions of cognitive, conative and affective dispositions, and a deeper analysis of these may be expected to lead to a comprehensive theory of cognition and with it a more coherent view than we at present have of the diverse series of mental adjustments which we denote by the term ' intelligence.'

By regarding the concept as a living growing mental entity I have been able elsewhere to frame such a theory of cognition,[1] and with the help of Prof. Stopford to show how this theory is congruous with observed phenomena of the neural basis of our minds, the cerebro-spinal nervous system.[2]

[1] *Elements in Thought and Emotion.*

[2] " The Neural Substrata of Reflective Thought," *Brit. Journal of Medical Psychology*, vol. v, pt. 2, 1925, and Chapter iv. in this book.

I present this view of the organic growth of the concept as a supplement to, and not at all as an alternative to, those mental processes which Prof. Spearman has set forth in his book on *Intelligence*. It presents perhaps a provisional attempt at what he desiderates under the phrase ' a mental cytology.'

Conclusions

The conclusions to which my studies during many years on this subject have led me are:

1. That the process of differentiation and progressive refinement which concepts undergo in man's brief span from childhood to age must be regarded not as a process of disintegration, but rather as one of organic growth.

2. That this growth is largely due to a selective activity which appropriates congruous mental material from the multitudinous data presented for selection in the continuity of the perceptual flux.

3. That this growth of concepts is one cause of the gradual modification which is observable in our cognitive dispositions and which results in what we colloquially call mental maturity.

4. That this growth may in some way be likened to that by which a biological organism attains a highly differentiated and diversified structure while still maintaining its original unity.

5. That the laws of this growth need to be determined by an extended course of experimental work and observation.

6. That this growth is one of the factors which go to make up that complex series of mental adjustments which together we call ' intelligence.'

7. That intelligence may tentatively and provisionally be defined as *the disciplined power of supplementing and refashioning the conceptual content of the mind by means of, or in response to, new perceptual experience.*

CHAPTER III

MEANING AND ERROR

In the problem of Meaning and Error, Epistemology, Logic, Psychology, and Etymology, all find an inevitable point of contact. It is necessary to go back little more than half a century to see something of the changes which have resulted in the present epoch of disintegration.

During the last half-century Bradley, in one chapter of his *Logic*, went far to demolish Associationism in Logic and Psychology, and in another the logic of a classification which is of fixed immobile particulars.[1]

In Epistemology, Alexander has more recently identified mental process with neural process.[2]

Psychology under the initiative of William James entered a phase in which it came to be

---

[1] " The dragons slain by our metaphysical St George (F. H. Bradley) were those of atomism and its allies in all their various forms. One famous chapter destroys associationism in logic and psychology ; another, the mechanical doctrine of the formal syllogism ; another, the logic of a classification which is of fixed, immobile particulars. Truth and reality are not to be looked for in any separate thing. ' The Truth is the whole ' " (" Spinoza in Recent English Thought," by L. Roth, *Mind*, vol. xxxvi, No. 142, April 1928).

[2] " We are forced, therefore, to go beyond the mere correlation of the mental with these neural processes and to identify them " (*Space, Time and Deity*, vol. ii, p. 5).

regarded as 'genetic,' yet James himself never fully realized the implications of this. Many years before his death he saw that the first step towards a synthesis of the complementary but diverse aspects of the psycho-neural problem lay in finding something in the nature of a single constituent element of our cognitive dispositions. " We seem," he wrote (1890), " if we are to have a psycho-neural law at all, thrust right back on something like the mental-atom theory, since the molecular fact being an element of the brain would seem naturally to correspond not to total thoughts but to elements of thought." [1] At the end of his life James attempted to find such a mental atom or constituent element of all our cognitions in the concept, but he was hampered in this quest by the traditional view of the concept, which regarded it as a static rigid entity which never varied. " A concept never varies," [2] he said in one of the chapters in his posthumously published volume on *Problems of Philosophy*. In this brief statement he was voicing the traditional philosophic view. Even genius, which often shows itself as a force working against the thought currents of its own time to produce new times, cannot wholly free itself from the traditions in which it has grown up.

Bergson saw that any attempt to explain thought

[1] *Textbook of Psychology*, p. 464.
[2] *Some Problems of Philosophy*, p. 53.

by means of rigid and unchanging elements was hopeless, and postulated a view of the concepts or mental symbols as "supple, mobile, almost fluid representations always ready to mould themselves on the fleeting forms of intuition." [1]

In a paper read before the British Association in 1928 [2] I showed reasons for the belief that the mental symbols which constitute our 'knowledge' are subject to a process of organic growth by the selective acquisition of new mental material from the multitudinous data presented for selection in the continuity of the perceptual flux. I traced in outline the growth of my own concept of a recent President of the British Association, Sir Arthur Keith, and showed that my present concept of him is the result of a growth-process extending over a period of twenty to twenty-five years. If this view be valid and be applicable to all the mental symbols of which our knowledge is composed, it will be seen to have obvious and direct bearing on the subject of 'meaning'; and the 'meaning' of any term will be seen to be the mental symbol or symbols which have by acquired and traditional usage become attached to it. If these mental symbols are subject to the growth process, they will obviously show great change in the onto-genetic phases of the individual life—the succes-

---

[1] *An Introduction to Metaphysics*, p. 18.
[2] "The Organic Growth of the Concept as One of the Factors in Intelligence," *British Journal of Psychology*, July, 1928.

sive periods in the intellectual growth of each of
our individual selves. Here we may find a partial
clue to the various logomachies which have been
dinned down to us through the ages. It follows,
too, that if from the standpoint of psychology we
may regard the mental symbols which go to make
up what we call our ' knowledge ' as subject to
such a process of organic growth—a growth in
mass or bulk accompanied by an ever-increasing
differentiation and refinement in structure—this
provides us with the psychological aspect or equivalent of the process which in Logic is called
' analysis,' and a mechanistic logic which is concerned mostly with terms will have to be replaced
by a humanistic science more congruous with the
living processes to which our mental symbols are
subject.

It would seem, then, from this preliminary consideration that we have living and growing mental
symbols to which are attached relatively static and
stable verbal symbols, and that these have a
relation to one another not unlike that which
obtains between living fruit-trees or rose-trees and
the labels attached to them to denote their several
varieties. As the trees pass through their processes
of seasonal growth, while the labels remain unchanged, so the various mental symbols which go
to make up what we call our knowledge also pass
through their processes of ontogenetic growth,

while the verbal symbols or terms which we use to denote them remain relatively stable and unchanged.

A consideration of the argument from the usage of what we call different ' languages ' reinforces this view. The combination of mental symbols which are called up by the phrase " Give me my hat " may just as readily be called up by the phrase " Donnez moi mon chapeau." And from the paucity of terms in language, or lack of their adequate diffusion, arises the commonplace experience which confronts us in any dictionary, where we learn that multitudinously different ' meanings ' or ' senses ' have in the long process of history become attached to different terms, or that quite different mental symbols are often denoted by the same verbal symbols. Yet the very ambiguity which arises from this disability is a happy factor in the permanent enrichment of our intellectual heritage. If, indeed, the fecundity of language were equal to the fecundity of thought, if it were as easy to invent and propagate new terms as to give birth to new ideas, and we were robbed of the power of using terms in different ' senses,' life itself would be deprived of one of its saving graces. Humour would suffer an inevitable decline. The pantomime lady would no longer be able to say, " You are treading on my *train*, and it is not intended to carry passengers! " and

Charles Lamb might never have remarked to the friend who sat down to whist with dirty hands, " My dear ——, if dirt were trumps, what *hands* you would have!" Literature thus shorn of much of its exquisite frolicsomeness would be in serious danger of becoming as dull as the jargon in a modern textbook of neurology.

The conclusion that the ' meanings ' of terms both severally and in their illimitable conjunctions and combinations consist in the mental symbols which a long usage has empirically come to attach to them, finds confirmation in the neurological studies which have been made during the past half-century of the differing conditions which have been found associated in intimate studies of aphasia.

A detailed consideration of this aspect of the subject would involve too much reference to technical neurology to justify its being considered fully here. Suffice it to say that it is now well recognized that this disability may involve:

(1) Impairment of the power of recognizing verbal symbols (*a*) by ear or (*b*) when written.

(2) The power of giving expression to these verbal symbols both (*a*) orally and (*b*) graphically.

(3) The loss of power of appreciation of the subtleties of the interaction of the mental symbols which are denoted by the terms attached to them.

And, in the various combinations of these different phases of the disorder, cases present themselves in which words may be recognized but the significance of their various combinations is lost. Reading may be possible, but not verbal formulation.

Thanks to the initiative and laborious studies of Sir Henry Head,[1] observations on cases of this kind open the way to far more intimate knowledge than we at present have of the neurological aspect of the relation and interaction of verbal symbols with the mental symbols which they denote.[2]

I have regarded the mental symbols which constitute our knowledge as subject to a process of organic growth extending often over prolonged periods, and during this process they are liable to an erratic growth which demands continual and persistent pruning. This erratic growth we call error. Each mental symbol or concept must be regarded as a mediation in ever-varying degree between what we call human truth and what we call human error, and during the growth-process may become either more true or more erroneous. Each concept may, in short, be a *mis*-conception,

[1] *Aphasia and Kindred Disorders of Speech* (Cambridge University Press), 1926, 2 vols.
[2] For an admirable summary of recent work and views on this subject, *vide Thought and the Brain*, by Henri Piéron, International Library of Psychology, etc. (Kegan Paul), 1927.

and when grouped or rationalized with other misconceptions may help to form what we call an obsession—a composite mental structure in which some of the various elements are permeated with various degrees and kinds of error, or in which the relative importance of the various component parts are presented in disproportion, and so productive of different kinds and degrees of falsification of the entire structure.[1] We all of us in turn, and for the most part throughout our lives, suffer from such obsessions, which only quite slowly become altered as time goes on by the constant rain of new impressions on various sense organs or receptors—the constant flow of what we call new experience. Under such influences the contents of our minds slowly change, and the error is either slowly eliminated or, on the other hand, becomes more stereotyped in the falsification of the obsession.

It is useless to attempt any definition of error until we possess some accepted definition of truth. The one may shade into the other by a sensibly continuous gradation, and we must perforce be at present content to regard it as a variation of our various mental symbols from those which a cultivated and accepted usage has come to attach to the terms which severally denote them. My con-

[1] Sir Thomas Browne's *Pseudodoxia* or *Vulgar Errors* is a classical example of the examination of such obsessions.

tention is that by regarding the mental symbols or concepts of which our knowledge is built up as living and growing subjective constructions, we can frame a psychological theory of knowledge which is wide enough to embrace the whole universe of human error, human illusion, and human self-deception—a theory which I have elsewhere shown in outline to be congruous with observed phenomena of the neural basis of our minds, the cerebro-spinal nervous system.[1]   It was towards such a theory that James was working at the time of his death, and it will be only by the formulation of such a theory and a realization of its relation in detail to the affective side of consciousness that Psychology can free itself from illogical inferences derived from pathological cases.

The conclusions to which my studies over many years have led me are:

1. That the mental symbols of which our knowledge is composed must in any system of genetic psychology be regarded as subject to a growth process in the several and successive ontogenetic phases of the individual mind.

2. That these living and growing mental symbols are severally denoted by relatively stable and

[1] *Elements in Thought and Emotion* (1923). "The Neural Substrata of Reflective Thought," *British Journal of Medical Psychology*, vol. v, pt. 2, 1925, and Chapter iv in this book.

static word symbols which the logicians call
' terms.'

3. That the living and growing mental
symbols (which have variously been called
ideas, concepts, presentations, representations,
images, etc.) are the ' meanings' which the
slowly interacting and cumulative influence of
etymology, logic, usage, and tradition have
attached to the terms which severally denote
them.

4. That the organic growth with structural
differentiation which takes place in these mental
symbols is the psychological aspect of what in
Logic is termed ' analysis.'

5. That these growing symbols are ineradicably
subjective and permeated with error, this error
becoming greater as the symbols tend to vary from
the cultivated and accepted usage of the terms
employed to denote them.

6. That such erroneous mental symbols may
become gradually linked into groups, and become
finally rationalized into obsessions.

7. That to regard knowledge as an integrated
aggregation of such living and growing subjective
symbols goes far to provide us with a psychological theory of knowledge wide enough to em-

brace the whole universe of human error, human illusion, and human self-deception.

8. That this view of knowledge can be shown to be congruous with observed phenomena of the neural basis of our minds, the cerebro-spinal nervous system.

CHAPTER IV

THE NEURAL SUB-STRATA OF REFLECTIVE THOUGHT [1]

Any attempt to unravel the workings of the neural substrata of reflective thought involves the presupposition that we possess some coherent view of the phenomena presented to us by reflective thought itself, and also that this view, whatever it may be, is one which is congruous with the workings of the neural processes with which it is proposed to try and establish for it a definite relationship; and further, any coherent view of the nature of reflective thought involves the whole question of epistemology and lies within the ambit of metaphysics.

The psycho-neural problem has thus a twofold aspect, the metaphysical and the neural, and to attempt any solution of the problem from one side only would be something like trying to explain the

[1] This chapter was written under the belief that it was to be a joint contribution with Prof. Stopford, with whom the neurological part of the argument was slowly matured over a period of many months, but on its completion Prof. Stopford thought that his contribution was insufficient to justify his name appearing as a joint author and the writer felt reluctantly obliged to acquiesce in its withdrawal. He desires to express his appreciation of the inexpressible value to him of the help thus given and his sincerest thanks for it. The material has been left in its original form and in its general tenor expresses the views of both.

normal ontogenetic development of any living being by the study of structure or function alone apart from their reactions on one another. Huxley said fifty-five years ago that the psycho-neural problem was " the metaphysical problem of problems." [1]   Wm. James more than forty years ago stated that its solution when it came would come in terms of metaphysics,[2] and Sir Charles Sherrington said in his Address to the British Association in 1922 that " it is to the psychologist that we must turn to learn in full the contribution made to the integration of the animal individual by mind," [3] and that " the how of the mind's connection with its bodily place seems still utterly enigma." [4]

Psychology when James wrote of it was supposed to deal with ' states of consciousness,' which seems to connect it definitely with metaphysics. In its later developments, as experimental psychology and psycho-physics it has become as inseparably connected with neurology, and however we may define it as a science *per se*, we may, for the purpose of the psycho-neural problem, regard it as a nexus between metaphysics on the one side and neurology on the other and as partaking in some degree of each. But in such a

[1] *On Sensation and Unity of Structure of the Sensiferous Organs.*
[2] *Text Book of Psychology*, p. 464.
[3] *Presidential Address, British Association*, 1922, p. 12.
[4] *Ibid.*, p. 15.

region of our knowledge—a region which is so largely inchoate and nebulous—words are, as Huxley once called them, only "noise and smoke," and may be left to the contentions of logomachists. It is only by an integration or synthesis of these diverse but complementary categories of knowledge and thought that a solution of the problem can be arrived at.

What we call man's knowledge may be said to consist of multitudinous mental symbols in ever-changing relations with one another—symbols which may be weighted with different kinds of what we usually call imagery—it may be visual, auditory, audito-motor, tactile or kinaesthetic, and which in the absence of any such characteristics are usually called ' abstract.' To these multitudinous symbols and their ever-changing inter-relations man has in the long course of his phylogenetic history affixed more or less empirically an equally multitudinous number of verbal symbols which we call ' names,' [1] and it has through the ages been one of the persistent functions of logic to induce cultivated man to abandon the primitive and youthful practice of attaching indiscriminately either a number of different names to the same mental symbol or a

---

[1] These ' names ' are subject to the same processes of error as the symbols which they denote, whether in their growth, structure or interpretation.

number of different mental symbols to the same name. Even the philosophers have not always complied with this behest of the logicians, and we find that these mental symbols, when regarded collectively, have in the past been variously denoted by the terms ' ideas,' ' concepts,' ' pre-sentations,' ' representations,' ' intuitions,' ' no-tions,' ' images,' etc. After Hume's death, and for the most part as the result of his writings, the English tradition more or less crystallized into the doctrine that the human mind was concerned with forming discrete ' ideas ' and making them cohere in accordance with certain laws of ' association.' ' The association of ideas ' was held to be the essential mental function. James' *Principles of Psychology* dealt this doctrine a heavy blow, and Bradley is held by some to have demolished it, but we imagine that Bradley himself might have been more inclined to regard the doctrine as a half-truth, which, like every other half-truth, is ever falling deeper and deeper into the pit of error the more it is regarded as a whole truth. James' *Principles* pointed to the primary continuity of mental life and showed that what first required explanation was not the method of effecting connections or ' associations ' but the growth of distinctions, both in " the big, blooming, buzzing confusion " of the immediate per-ceptual flux and also in the continuity of

the trains of thought which are unceasingly
passing through what we colloquially call our
' minds.'

We propose to follow the tradition of Wm.
James in using for these mental symbols generally,
whatever type of imagery be connected with
them or whether they be entirely abstract, the
term ' Concepts.' This term concept, which goes
back to Plato, has long denoted in philosophical
discourse a mental entity having in philosophic
parlance the characteristics of concreteness, univer-
sality and invariability. Many years before his
death James saw that the first step towards a
synthesis of the complementary but diverse aspects
of the psycho-neural problem lay in finding something in the nature of a single constituent element
of our cognitive dispositions. " We seem," he
wrote (1890), " if we are to have an elementary
psycho-physic law at all thrust right back on
something like the mental-atom theory since the
molecular fact being an element of the brain
would seem naturally to correspond not to total
thoughts but to elements of thought." [1] At the
end of his life James attempted to find such a
mental atom or constituent element of all our
cognitions in the concept, but he was hampered
in this quest by the traditional view of the concept
which regarded it as a static rigid entity which

---

[1] *Textbook of Psychology*, p. 464.

E

never varied. " A concept never varies,"[1] he said in one of the chapters in his posthumously published volume on Problems of Philosophy. In this brief statement he was voicing the traditional philosophic view.

Bergson saw that any attempt to explain thought by means of rigid and unchanging elements was hopeless, and in his *Introduction to Metaphysics* postulated a view of the concept or mental symbol as a supple, mobile, almost fluid representation always ready to mould itself on the fleeting forms of intuition.[2] This view of Bergson has recently been elaborated by one of us (G. G. C.), with the aid of Mr Santayana, and he shows by a number of concrete examples[3] that a concept when once formed grows in the course of the ontogenetic life process in a somewhat similar fashion to the different organs of the body by a growth in mass or bulk accompanied by progressive differentiation of structure. This view of the concept satisfies the requirements of James and Bergson and pro-

---

[1] *Some Problems of Philosophy*, p. 53.

[2] " Certainly, concepts are necessary to metaphysics for all the other sciences work as a rule with concepts, and metaphysics cannot dispense with the other sciences. But it is only truly itself when it goes beyond the concept, or at least when it frees itself from rigid and ready-made concepts in order to create a kind very different from those which we habitually use ; I mean supple, mobile and almost fluid representations, always ready to mould themselves on the fleeting forms of intuition." *An Introduction to Metaphysics*, by Henri Bergson ; translation by T. E. Hulme, p. 18.

[3] *Elements in Thought and Emotion*, chap. ii, on Percept and Concept.

vides us with a mental element subject to continual modification by means of the new experience which is being progressively acquired through sense-perception—an element of which all our cognitions may be held to be gradually built up in the course of the ontogenetic life process. We adopt this term ' concept ' in the sense and with the connotations here noted as the term by which we denote the symbol or mental atom of which James thirty-five years ago indicated the need, and we proceed to enquire what this mental element of our various and multitudinous cognitions has as its correlate in the neural elements and processes of the brain.

During the twenty years before his death the late Richard Semon of Vienna in laborious biological studies of the abiding effects of transient stimuli on irritable living tissues—studies which he pursued through a wide range of biological types culminating in Man—gave to the abiding effects of such stimuli the term ' engram.' In the last of his works, *Bewusstseinsvorgang und Gehirnprozess*, published in 1920, he considers more intimately the engram in relation to the psychoneural problem, and in this connection he means by it a physiological pattern established by successive stimuli and resulting in a condition in which there have gradually been produced, by recurrent stimuli and faciliation, paths for a ready connection of neural impulse between many and diversely scattered groups of neurones in various cerebral areas. These engrams when once formed may remain in a latent condition or may at any time become active by an impulse discharged through them. In the arrangement of terms which Semon adopted, the ' engram ' remained in a latent condition until ' ecphorized ' or made active by the discharge of a neural impulse through it. These engrams were held by him to exist in all degrees of complexity, to dichotomize again and again, and at each period of their active or ' ecphorized ' condition to form new engrams within themselves.[1] It is further to be noted that Semon regarded the mental correlates of the engrams (or the symbols which we call ' concepts ') to be below the ' threshold of consciousness ' during the latent condition of the engram and as above the threshold during its active or ' ecphorized ' condition. We are inclined to regard this as an inadequate explanation of this phenomenon and shall refer to the point again later.

We find in studying the masterly paper by Drs Head and Holmes on " Sensory Disturbances from Cerebral Lesions " [2] that some at any rate of Semon's conclusions had been also reached by these investigators, although the terms in which

[1] *Mnemic Psychology*, by Richard Semon, p. 258.
[2] *Brain*, vol. xxxiv, p. 183.

their conclusions are expressed differ in the way which is usual when workers in the same field of research are engaged on the same problem but working in isolation from one another. This classic piece of research was immediately concerned only with those groups of sensory impulses which reach the brain through the spinal cord and medulla, but we consider that the conclusions reached in regard to the slowly-acquired systems of paths in the cortex for these sensory impulses have a much wider and more universal application, and that it will be only by their application to all the afferent nerves of the cerebro-spinal system, and perhaps also to the sympathetic and para-sympathetic systems that their full significance will be realized and the contribution which they, with Semon's engrams, make to a solution of the psycho-neural problem will be fully understood.

Their researches led them to the conclusion that sensory impulses from the cord and medulla, after exciting the essential thalamic centres, leave the optic thalami in five main functional groups for distribution in the cortex: [1]

1. Those which underlie postural recognition and the appreciation of passive movement.

2. Those which underlie the recognition of tactile differences or the power of appreciating

[1] *Ibid.*

those qualities of touch other than contact and roughness (*e.g.* weights of objects on hand).

3. Those upon which depend spacial discrimination (compass points) and its allied faculty, the recognition of size and shape.

4. Those impulses which enable the patient to recognize the spot stimulated (localization).

5. Thermal impulses.

They show that the appreciation and recognition of the import of these groups of sensory impulses depend on separate ' schemata ' or systems of neural paths slowly formed during the ontogenetic life process and which may be severally destroyed by cortical lesions. These ' schemata ' along which such impulses pass enable us to recognize, locate and analyse, with an accuracy so subtle as to be utterly beyond expression by means of the clumsy machinery of language, the results of sensory impulses which cannot be resolved into types of imagery and yet which contribute in most important ways to our integrated experience. They have their correlates in our conceptual knowledge but with a refinement and subtlety which often eludes description. In the arrangement of terms adopted by Drs Head and Holmes the ' focus of attention ' sweeps over these neural schemata which " modify the impressions produced by incoming sensory impulses in such a way that the final sensations of position or locality rise into consciousness charged with a relation to something that has happened before. Destruction of such schemata by a lesion of the cortex renders impossible all recognition of position or of the locality of a stimulated spot on the affected part of the body."[1]

Making the necessary allowances for various conditions under which investigators working separately in the same research field, at the same time, will obviously precipitate their conclusions by means of different terms we seem driven inevitably to the conclusion that the neural 'schemata' of Drs Head and Holmes are identical with Semon's neural 'engrams,' and the psychological abstraction which we call the 'focus of attention' has as its neural correlate that part of the entire 'engrammic' or 'schematic' system which is endowed at any particular moment with the highest neural potential, and the shifting in the engrammic or schematic system of the point of highest neural potential is the physiological correlate of the movement of the 'focus of attention.'

From our present point of view it seems necessary for us to invert this statement. From the biological standpoint it seems to us that in the course of the ontogenetic life process there has

[1] " Sensory Disturbances from Cerebral Lesions," *Brain*, vol. xxxiv, p. 189.

gradually been formed in response to the lifelong aggregation of the effects of sensory impulses a huge and complicated network of physiological paths in which are enmeshed innumerable neurones in various parts of the cerebral organs. These physiological paths were termed by Semon ' engrammic systems ' and by Drs Head and Holmes neural ' schemata.' We hold that along this huge system of paths, and partly as the result of fresh sensory stimuli, neural impulses are being continually propagated now in one part of the system now in another; that a neural impulse activating one part of the system tends to activate both adjacent and subjacent parts; that those parts which are in a sufficient state of activity tend to throw above the threshold of consciousness their psychological correlates; and that the part of the system which is at any moment most active owing to the intensity of its neural potential is the part which forms the neural correlate of the psychological abstraction which introspective psychologists and even at times behaviourists call the ' focus of attention.' [1]

[1] In addition to what psychologists call the ' focus of attention ' there is, of course, also the accompanying condition for which James used the term ' fringe of consciousness.' We think that the condition denoted by this term has in part as its neural correlate those regions of an active engrammic system where the neural potential is lower than in the track of the main impulse. It is amongst the commonplaces of our everyday experience that any particular part of, for example, an extended visual image in the field of perception may be at one moment in the ' focus of attention ' and at another moment in the ' fringe of

Here then in the ' concept ' and the ' engram ' (or schema) we seem to have the related thought elements and neural elements which are indispensable for any synthetic or synoptic view of the thought processes on the one side and the neural processes on the other—of thought regarded as a psychological quality of the human mind and the neurological processes which accompany it and furnish its neural correlates. The concept or thought element is the abiding result of a long process of growth or building-up from the acquired results of sense-perception, an element which is subject to unceasing change in response to new sense stimuli, and growing with a growth characterized by an increase in mass accompanied by progressive differentiation of structure. On the neural side as the anatomical and physiological correlate of the concept we have the ' engram ' of Semon or the neural ' schema ' of Drs Head

consciousness,' and that the change from one to the other is under the control of what we usually call ' volition.' Here at once rise two fundamental questions into neither of which we at present propose to enter :

(1) What are the neural correlates of the psychological abstraction which we call volition ?

(2) What are the functional relations in an act of visual perception of the stimuli (*a*) from the macula, and (*b*) from other parts of the retina ?

The first of these questions seems to us beyond the present bounds of scientific speculation, and its solution must be contingent on our interpretation of the term ' volition.' The answer to the second question is probably within the knowledge of Sir Grafton Elliot Smith who has made this subject peculiarly his own.

and Holmes consisting of a slowly formed physiological pattern between groups of neurones in different areas of the brain, this pattern also being in continual process of modification and growth like the concept of which we hold it to be the neural correlate. Each psychological entity in thought, each mental symbol or concept, has, we think, its neural engram, each of these minor engrams forming a small integral part of much larger engrammic or schematic systems.

These slowly acquired neural paths may be at one time latent and at another time active, or to use Semon's term ' ecphorized,' owing to the discharge of a neural impulse through them. What is known in the jargon of the day as ' the subconscious mind ' has in our view as its neural correlate the multitudinous systems of engrams slowly formed during the entire ontogenetic life process, these engrams being in a latent as distinguished from an active condition. And the ' act of recall ' to consciousness, be it total or partial, of the multitudinous mental symbols and their inter-relations has its neural correlate in the activating of those parts of the entire engrammic or schematic systems which form the neural correlates of the groups of inter-related concepts which are being for the moment ' recalled ' to consciousness.

Just as a concept grows in response to the sensory

impulses which form an integral part of the perceptual processes by a growth in bulk or mass
accompanied by progressively increasing differentiation of structure, so too with the engram. The
sensory impulses from the receptor organs which
during the ontogenetic life process are continually
changing it from a latent to an active condition
lead to a growth by which its neural paths are
being continually enlarged by ramification and by
an increasing number of neurones being functionally incorporated in it, and in these kindred processes of growth in the concept and the engram
we have examples of that power of modification
and adjustment which on the biological side is
usually called ' adaptation to environment ' and
on the mental or psychological side is one form of
what is usually called ' intelligence.'

This view seems to us to open the way to a
physiological explanation of what we call ' memory ' to complement the work which has been
carried out by psychologists on the psychological
aspect of this subject. The ' distributed repetitions ' of the psychologists have in our view as
their neural correlates the activation at similarly
distributed intervals of the same engrammic systems. These engrammic or schematic systems
may be held to become more permanently established by what the physiologists call ' facilitation '
when their periods of activation are suitably ' dis-

tributed ' than is possible by a single period or more rapidly successive periods of activation, and if such engrammic or schematic systems are allowed to remain latent for an indefinite period all power of reviving them may disappear, and result in a permanent ' forgetfulness.'

But it is of the essence of what we call ' memory ' that the subject matter involved should be capable of being ' recalled ' by some agency other than the peripheral receptor organs by means of which it was originally acquired—that the engrammic systems which in the acquirement of the subject-matter were largely formed by successive series of sensory impulses from the receptor organs, should, for the purpose of ' memory,' be capable of being activated by a central agency apart from the receptor organs, and we think that this will be found to be one of the functions of the Optic Thalami.

To the essential organs of the thalami Drs Head and Holmes assigned the function of being in some way the centre of consciousness for the affective side of sensation. If these investigators are right, and we accept their conclusions on this point, then it seems to us that to these organs we may assign a part, by means of some form of conditioned reflexes, in furnishing the affective elements which enter into every act of perception. It is well recognized that every such act involves

the commingling and interaction of old knowledge with the new which is being acquired in
that act of perception. " For in a perception, as
James said, half comes to us from the thing per-
ceived and half out of our own heads." [1] This
would seem to involve the activation of engrams
from within as well as by sensory impulses from
without, of stimulation from a central source as
well as stimulation from the peripheral receptor
organs. `We hold that it is a part of the function
of the essential organs of the thalami to provide
this central stimulation; that in the processes
of perception there is usually an activation of
the engrams from the essential thalamic organs
supplemented by activation from the peripheral
receptor organs, and that these two series of impulses, internal from the essential thalamic organs
and external from the peripheral receptor organs,
furnish together the ' a priori data ' and the ' sense
data ' involved in every act of perception. In
this activation of any group or system of engrams
by the essential thalamic organs we find also the
neural correlate of that condition which is known

---

[1] " The Artistry of Truth," by Prof. S. Alexander, *Hibbert Journal*,
January, 1925, p. 303.
" As it lies in your fancy, then, this object, the reality, is a complex
and elusive entity, the sum at once and the residuum of all particular
impressions which, underlying the present one, have bequeathed to it
their surviving linkage in discourse and consequently endowed it with
a large part of its present character " (*The Life of Reason*, by G. Santayana, i, p. 82).

to psychologists as ' pre-perception,' and in the
changeful continuity of this neural process by
which different engrams or schemata become successively activated without stimulation from the
peripheral receptor organs we find the neural correlate of what is usually called ' reverie ' and also
of a large part of the mental processes, which fall
within the range of what we call ' ratiocination.'

   But in ' memory,' in ' reverie,' and in ' ratiocination,' it is often of the essence of the process
that we should be able, as we say, to roll a subject
over and over in what we colloquially call our
' minds,' and survey different parts and aspects of
it in continually changing and alternating processes of succession; and we hold that the neural,
correlates of these various mental processes are
intimately bound up with the functions of the
paths which return from the various parts of the
cortex to the optic thalami—the cortico-thalamic
paths.   It is little material to the primary question
of the function of these paths whether they return
from all parts of the cortex (Head and Holmes)
or only from parts other than the association areas
(Bianchi).   This is a question which neurology
has not perhaps yet been finally able to determine.
It is one of the many questions for the future.   But
a current view of the function of these paths is
that they are concerned in transmitting impulses
by which the cortex is enabled to exercise in some

way a control over the functioning of the thalami.

It is part of our thesis to offer an alternative view of the function of these paths and we suggest that they are return paths for reflex neural impulses from the cortex which excite relay cells in the thalami, and that these relay cells in turn send stimuli both to the essential thalamic organs and also to the same cortical areas from which the paths conveying the return impulse originated. We think that in this way a multitudinous series of complex conditioned reflexes become established the end of which is to provide a means by which a continual circulation of neural impulse may be maintained without stimulation from the peripheral receptor organs—a circulation which enables any series of engrams or schemata to be continuously activated and their psychological correlates or concepts, in their ever-changing relations, kept continuously above the threshold of consciousness and alternated in the various ways which are a condition of reflective thought.

Merely to state this view is to raise at once the whole complicated question of the nature of what we call 'inhibition.' It would carry us beyond the purview of our subject to discuss this question in any detail. We merely note that the term is applied alike (1) to the diminished heart beat resulting from stimulation of the vagus, (2) to the diminished secretion of glands under certain conditions of the sympathetic and para-sympathetic systems, (3) to the diminished activity under certain conditions of some neural organs, and (4) to phases in the processes of the reciprocal innervation of the opposed muscular groups controlling the skeletal framework.

We take it that the term as usually employed connotes an active or positive neural impulse which *diminishes* certain kinds of physiological action, and in this sense we think that as applied to a hypothetical restraining action on the thalami by the cortex, and to the reciprocal innervation of opposed muscular groups, it will in the end prove to have been logically inadmissible. We find it stated in works of physiology that although no inhibitory mechanism has been discovered in skeletal muscles, and although there is no known instance of a peripheral nerve which when stimulated causes relaxation of these muscles, yet the fact that an extensor muscle severed from its distal attachment lengthens when the flexion reflex is stimulated is held to prove the existence of an *active* inhibitory process. We hold this to be an illogical inference which will in due time be eliminated by the application of Occam's razor. *Entia non sunt multiplicanda praetor necessitatem*, and we see no necessity for postulating the existence of a special inhibitory mechanism to explain this phenomenon: we see only the need of postulating a neural mechanism capable of simultaneously diminishing the stimuli to one group of muscles and increasing those to the opposed group, thus securing a co-ordinated and simultaneous intensive adjustment of the neural potential supplying both flexors and extensors. We adopt in short a view something like that expressed by Professor Bianchi in his book on *The Mechanism of the Brain and the Function of the Frontal Lobes*, viz. that what is usually called ' inhibition ' must in many cases be regarded more as a change in neural potential than as the manifestation and result of a special inhibitory mechanism, unless indeed this so-called inhibitory mechanism be regarded as one which acts by re-directing or changing the intensity of the neural potential. Whether future research will confirm Professor Bianchi's opinion that all inhibition is a re-direction of neural potential remains for the future to determine, but we suggest that a similar kind of neural mechanism, whatever it may be, will be found at work effecting the intensive and directional changes of neural impulse in the cerebral engrammic or schematic systems and also those involved in reciprocal muscular innervation.

We regard then as one of the factors contributing to the neural sub-strata of reflective thought the formation during the ontogenetic life process

F

of innumerable engrams extending from the thalami to the various cortical lobes connected with their respective receptor organs, visual, auditory, olfactory, tactile, etc.: that these engrams intercommunicate through the association areas; and that, however complex may be their structure and however extended their distribution and range, they each comprise a neural mechanism which, by means of a series of conditioned reflexes, can maintain a continuous circulation of neural impulse between the thalami and the cortex: we think that these multitudinous engrammic or schematic systems may be activated either (1) from the essential organs of the thalami, or (2) from the peripheral receptor organs, or (3) concurrently from both these sources, and that by some means at present beyond our knowledge the neural impulse whether from the thalami or the receptor organs or from both may be under a continual process of re-direction to different parts of the entire aggregate of engrammic systems.

" The sensory cortex is the storehouse of past impressions, "[1] and these engrams which are the outcome of the ontogenetic life process come doubtless to incorporate in their systems the multitudinous neurones found in the different layers of the cortex; and in the unimaginable intricacy

[1] " Sensory Disturbances from Cerebral Lesions," by Henry Head and Gordon Holmes, *Brain*, vol. xxxiv, p. 189.

and complexity of the multitudinous paths formed by means of these cells and by the varying resistances offered by the synapses between them there is we think gradually built up and stabilized the neural counterpart of what we retain of these past experiences.

In the stratified arrangement of the multitudinous neurones in the cortex and the diverse complexities of the engrams embracing the neurones in these different strata we see the neural mechanism involved in ' Generalization,' in ' Classification ' and in ' Abstraction ': in the ' Universals ' and ' Particulars ' of the Philosophers, in the ' Genera ' and ' Species ' of the Logicians and Biologists and in logical constructions like the ' Tree of Porphyry.' " Are genera and species," said Huxley, "realities or abstractions?" Viewed from the standpoint we are now presenting we think we must tentatively answer that they are abstractions.

We have already expressed the opinion that in the activation of engrams by the essential organs of the thalami will be found the neural correlates of a large part of the mental processes concerned in what we call ' ratiocination '; and in the results of the reciprocal interaction of the internal stimuli from these organs and the external stimuli from the peripheral receptor organs will we think be found the neural correlates of what the logicians call 'judgments.' Of such judgments we may take as a simple illustration the case of someone pointing to a rose and saying. " This rose is red! " Here we think there comes into play that condition which psychologists call ' pre-perception ': that this involves the partial activation by the essential thalamic organs of a large number of engrams—of the whole series of engrams which in the aggregate form the neural correlates of the mental symbol or concept ' rose ' and all its several differentiæ which happen to be stored in the cognitive dispositions of the person expressing the judgment; and that the sensory impulses from the peripheral receptor organ (the eye), simultaneously re-enforcing the internal stimuli from the essential thalamic organs to the engram which forms the neural correlate of the concept ' red,' furnishes the combination of neural processes which forms the neural correlate of, and which issues in, the judgment. And in logical judgments dealing with a greater number and a greater complexity of phenomena—judgments which we call ' considered judgments ': judgments which are not immediate but which are mediated by a discursive mental process—we consider that essentially the same neural processes will be found to be involved despite their greater complexity. Here we think is a suggestive theme to occupy the united attention of the logicians and the neurologists.

One of us (G. G. C.) has shown reasons from the psychological side for thinking that all the usual mental processes which we call observation, inference, imagination, reason, etc., can be resolved into the reactions and interactions of ' percepts ' and ' concepts ':[1] percepts being in his arrangement of terms the psychological correlates of the interactions of fresh sensory impulses from the various kinds of receptor organs with the processes of the organized neural tissues which are the outcome of the ontogenetic life process. If, throughout his argument we substitute for the psychological term ' concept ' the neural term ' engram ' or ' schema,' as denoting its neural correlate, the relation of the views expressed in this paper with his theory of epistemology will become at once apparent.

We have sketched now the more fundamental considerations upon which in our opinion depends a solution of that part of the psycho-neural problem which is concerned with reflective thought, and these considerations seem to bring us to the following conclusions.

Conclusions

1. We adopt the view of the concept postulated by Bergson and elaborated by Santayana and Campion as the psychological or mental element

[1] *Elements in Thought and Emotion.*

or atom desiderated and sought by Wm. James
as the first step towards the formulation of an
elementary psycho-physic law.   This provides
an element—largely the abiding, organized
and cumulative effects of sense-perception—
of which all our cognitions are gradually built
up during man's brief span from infancy to
age.

2. We have shown that the growth of this
mental element in its various manifestations is
congruous with the neurological processes which
establish in the course of the ontogenetic life
history physiological paths for impulses between
the multitudinous neurones in different lobes and
areas of the brain.   We adopt Semon's term
' engrams ' to denote these physiological paths and
Head's term ' neural schema ' as a permissible
synonym.   We regard the ' engram ' as the neural
correlate of the ' concept ' and the latent condition of the engram as the condition which usually
subsists when its conceptual correlate is ' below
the threshold of consciousness,' and the active or
' ecphorized ' condition of the engram as the condition which usually subsists when its conceptual
correlate is ' above the threshold of consciousness.'
But we think that this is only restrictedly true
and that it must be held to be merely one of a
larger complex of factors.   It is often we think
possible for an engram to be in an active or

'ecphorized' condition without its conceptual correlate becoming above the threshold of consciousness. We consider that herein may be found the explanation of those psycho-pathic states which are characterized by what are usually known as 'suppressed' phases of past experience. In these cases we think that the engrams which form the correlates of the suppressed experience may have become functionally dissociated from larger engrammic systems and especially from direct communication with the essential thalamic centres, and that it is their dissociated functioning which gives rise to the symptoms which are known to be associated with such suppressed phases of past experience.

3. We regard the aggregation of the 'engrammic systems' of neural paths when in a latent condition, *i.e.* when no impulse is passing through them, as the neural correlate of what is called 'the subconscious mind.'

4. We consider that just as a concept itself is changing by a process of growth in the way described during the life process of the individual this is accompanied by and has its neural correlate in a corresponding growth in the 'engram,' and that just as in our processes of active thought that quality which we call our 'attention' is transferred rapidly from concept to concept in all their

wide relations and through an unending series, so also is this associated with a corresponding change in the correlative pattern of neural impulse in the attendant ' engrams.'

5. We note and emphasize the fact which neurological science has brought to light within the last half-century that all afferent nerve stimuli in the cerebro-spinal nervous system pass into the optic thalami on their way both to the essential organs of the thalami and to the various cortical areas of the brain.

6. We adopt the view of Head and Holmes that the thalami form the great junctions where the afferent stimuli from all the receptor organs may be redistributed.   This function of the thalami as a great junction for afferent stimuli provides we think the neural mechanism by which the perception of touch through one of the fingers may be the means of exciting, *e.g.* what are called ' visual images,' by means of the optic lobes.

7. We adopt the view of Head and Holmes that the essential organs of the thalami perform in some way the function of the central seat of consciousness for the affective side of sensation and the cortex the seat of the discriminative perceptions of space, form, colour, sound, position, etc.

8. We regard the essential thalamic organs as affording by some form of conditioned reflexes

one means of activating the various engrammic systems, and alternatively that such activation may be the result of stimuli from the peripheral receptor organs or concurrently from both of these sources.

9. We regard that part of an active engrammic system in which the neural potential is most intense and which is in most direct communication with the essential thalamic organs as the neural correlate of what the psychologists call the ' focus of attention ' and those parts of the same active engrammic system in which the neural potential is less or which are in less direct communication with the essential thalamic organs as the neural correlate of what the psychologists call the ' fringe of consciousness.' But this in itself is in our opinion inadequate to explain all the associated phenomena which require for their full elucidation further research in the physiology of special sensation.

10. We regard the activation of the various engrammic systems by the essential thalamic organs as the neural process involved in what is usually called ' memory ' and in what Semon called the ' mnemic excitation ' (as distinguished from the original excitation) which ' ecphorizes ' the multitudinous engrams, changing them from a latent to an active condition, so bringing above the

'threshold of consciousness' the multitudinous and ever-changing concepts of which the 'engrams' form the neural correlates. We also regard this activation of engrams by the essential thalamic organs as furnishing the neural correlates of what in the chaotic vocabulary of our present discords, have been variously termed 'the datum' of consciousness, the '*a priori* data' of the perceptual processes and 'pre-perception.'

11. We regard the fibres which descend from the cortex to the thalami as conveying stimuli from the engrams in the various areas of localized perceptions or cognitive dispositions, and that these stimuli excite relay cells in the thalami which again send stimuli to the same cortical areas and that the continual action of this circulatory system of neural impulse from cortex to thalami and from thalami to cortex goes far to constitute the thalami as organs contributing in important ways to the continuity of reflective thought.

12. With the concept as an element of thought on the psychological side having the characteristics described and the engram as described by Semon furnishing its neural correlate; the first of these entities being infinitely mobile and ever in course of merging into others; and this mobility having as its neural correlate an ever-

shifting range of activation in an otherwise latent aggregate of engrammic systems, we seem to possess a view of complementary processes, psychological and neural, congruous with one another and affording together the needful explanation of the continuity and fluidity of thought. As to the processes by which the requisite changes in the direction of the neural potential are being constantly made we are unable at present to offer any hypothesis, but we imagine that when these are discovered they will be found somewhat similar to the processes which direct, alternate and adjust with finely graded and continually changing intensity the stimuli to the nerves supplying the balanced groups of muscles which alternately flex and extend the limbs.

13. These views seem logically to bring us to the conclusion that it is necessary for us to regard what is usually called ' inhibition ' as being, at any rate in some cases, more in the nature of a re-direction or intensive modification of neural potential than the effects of a positive neural discharge inhibiting other neural discharges. In this we find ourselves in agreement with the opinions expressed by Bianchi in his book on *The Mechanism of the Brain and the Function of the Frontal Lobes*, and by Morley Roberts in his book on *Warfare in the Human Body*,[1] but we realize that this

---

[1] *Op. cit.* chap. iv, " Inhibition and the Cardiac Vagus."

conclusion questions a current view of the inter-relation of cortical and thalamic functionings. We think that the implications involved in the phrase ' cortical control ' need to be further investigated and the attendant phenomena possibly re-inter-preted.

14. We regard the formation and functional maintenance of the multitudinous engrammic systems as the neural mechanism involved in the storage of past experience.

15. We regard the formation of complex en-grams embracing several or all of the various layers or strata of neurones in the cortex as pro-viding the neural mechanism involved in the mental processes of abstraction, generalization and classification.

16. We regard the concurrent activation of such engrams by both the essential thalamic organs and the various kinds of receptor organs as the neural processes concerned in immediate logical judgments and also in those mediated by a discursive mental process.

17. These views seem to us to open the way directly or indirectly to further research in the direction of

(a) A physiological explanation of ' memory ' to complement the work which has been done by psychologists during the last half century on the psychological aspect of this subject;

(*b*) A more specific application of the biologist's Recapitulation Theory to the mental development of Man;

(*c*) A closer investigation of the neural mechanism of sleep;

(*d*) An investigation of the neural mechanism of ' suppression,' ' dissociation,' ' conflict,' and ' psychological inversion,' and

(*e*) A study concurrently both psychological and neural of the phenomena of human error and self-deception, a subject which the great philosophic system makers have more or less tended to ignore, yet one which must form an important part of the prolegomena to any really philosophic theory of the state.

In presenting this outline of our subject and these conclusions we are fully conscious that many may think we have strayed too far over the boundary line between science and speculation and suffered the stream of our argument to become not a little contaminated by mixture with what some will regard as the turbid waters of metaphysics.[1]   If this be so we may recall two sayings

[1] " When we talk of ' psychology as a natural science,' we must not assume that that means a sort of psychology that stands at last on solid ground. It means just the reverse : it means a psychology particularly fragile, and into which the waters of metaphysical criticism leak at

of Thomas H. Huxley: (1) that " the sensory operations have been, from time immemorial, the battle-ground of philosophers,"[1] and (2) that " metaphysical speculation follows as closely on physical theory as black care upon the horseman."[1] Yet in these views we seem to reach a further stage on the pathway which will lead ultimately to a resolution of the diverse biological processes which underlie the relation of the abstraction which we call ' consciousness ' to the neural parts and processes which furnish its anatomical and physiological sub-strata. But the dark Psyche of the Greeks will ever remain dark to the investigations of mortal man. The utmost we can do is to unravel little by little the physiological and biochemical processes by means of which the Psyche works and correlate these processes with the various neural organs in which they have their seat and through which they perform their functions.

It was forty-five years ago that Huxley declared the psycho-neural problem to be " the metaphysical problem of problems "; and, to go still further back than Huxley and to a complementary view, if Kant was right that the constitution of our minds pre-

every joint, a psychology all of whose elementary assumptions and data must be reconsidered in wider connections and translated into other terms." *Textbook of Psychology*, by Wm. James, p. 467.

[1] *On Sensation and the Unity of Structure of the Sensiferous Organs.* (1879.)

determines the form which all our knowledge takes, then we think that to some such working of the neural vehicle of thought which we have outlined must be ascribed its part in all the ratiocinations of the philosophers, in all the refinements of the theologians, in the creations of the poets, the painters, the sculptors and the musicians, in the uttermost particles of the physicists and in the artistic abstractions of the mathematicians. The Newtonian method of analysis and subsequent synthesis will then be found not merely to be applicable to mental science but to be itself actually conditioned by the mode of working of the neural processes which underlie that science, and which furnish the sub-strata of all the phenomena amongst which we live and move and have our being.

It will be obvious that in a subject of such complexity, upon the study of which philosophy and science can hardly as yet be said to have fully entered, any theory or hypothesis at present put forward can at best be merely provisional, and will perhaps attain its most useful end by directing attention to a method of approaching the subject which, whatever its defects as here set forth, possesses at least the merit of recognizing that it will be only by considering synoptically and finding an integration of both sides of the problem— psychological and neural—that any real success in its solution is likely to be achieved. And, in view of what Mr Santayana has happily termed " the many sided ignorance " to which in these days individuals are all reduced, it would seem that it will lie with workers in the diverse spheres of metaphysics, logic, psychology, neurology and even wider ranges of biology to test in every possible way the view here outlined, to supply its myriad needs of detail and to refashion it where faulty by means of the new light which will be shed upon it by our ever increasing knowledge. We believe that study on these lines, directed rigorously to the pursuit of truth will lead ultimately to an outlook on man not essentially different from that envisioned by the sages and seers of all historic times.

CHAPTER V

THE THALAMO-CORTICAL [1] CIRCULATION OF NEURAL IMPULSE

In Chapter IV I arrived at the conclusion that the neural paths which descend from different parts of the cortex to the thalami—the cortico-thalamic paths—are concerned, not with providing means for the exercise of direct and positive inhibitory influence over the thalami, but with the maintenance of a circulation of neural impulse between the thalami and the cortex.

Further consideration has made it seem apparent to me that the conception of a thalamo-cortical circulation of neural impulse will in the future come to be found as fundamental for the neurology of what we colloquially call ' thought ' as the conception of a circulation of the blood is for modern physiology! This view will doubtless, at first, appear to many as fantastic as did

[1] I am much indebted to Sir Grafton Elliot Smith for this term. I had written to him about what I then called the *cortico-thalamic* circulation, etc. In his reply he inverted my term and referred to *thalamo-cortical* relations. This was, from my own point of view, so great and manifest an improvement that I wish gratefully to acknowledge my indebtedness to him for it, as well as for much corrective and creative criticism of the chapter as a whole. To Prof. Stopford I am also indebted for much similar and valuable help, and also in the construction of the diagrams so admirably drawn by Miss Davison.

that of the circulation of the blood over 300 years
ago when Harvey first propounded it; and just
as that view, though generally accepted during
Harvey's later life, was only finally established
after his death and with the aid of the subsequently
invented microscope, so the hypothesis of a
thalamo-cortical circulation of neural impulse can,
if correct, only be established by a process of in-
duction extending over a long period of years and
into, or even perhaps through, another generation.

Many of the anatomical facts about the vascular
system were intimately known before their method
of functioning was demonstrated by Harvey.
Many anatomical facts as to the cerebral organs
are known to-day, but a large generalization as
to their co-ordinated functioning in reflective
thought has still to be widely accepted. And as
the doctrine of the circulation of the blood gave
functional coherence to a mass of previously discovered facts about the vascular system, so the
hypothesis of a thalamo-cortical circulation of
neural impulse must also, if correct, be expected
to give functional coherence both to the large
number of facts which have been accumulated as
to cortical localization, to the neurological aspect
of the multitudinously varied phenomena of ordinary mental life, and also to those which are associated with pathological and traumatic varieties of
aphasia.

The path by which I reached this conclusion was long and tedious. It began nearly forty years ago with a study of what psychologists have for years denoted by the phrase 'cognitive dispositions.' How and of what elements are our cognitive dispositions constituted? This question resulted in an intimate study of this aspect of psychology at the point where Wm. James left it at the conclusion of his later and briefer course. In the final chapter of this book he says: " We seem, if we are to have an elementary psycho-physic law at all, thrust right back upon something like the mental atom theory, for the molecular fact, being an element of the brain, would seem naturally to correspond not to total thoughts but to elements of thought." [1]

Nineteen years later the publication of his posthumous work, *Some Problems of Philosophy*, showed that he had been trying to find in the ' concept ' that element of thought or mental atom which he had postulated many years before, and to read the chapters in this book dealing with " Percept and Concept " is to be able to realize how much he was hampered in this quest by the traditional philosophic view of the concept which regarded it as a ' universal '—a static stable mental entity which never varied. " Particular facts decay and our perceptions of them vary. A con-

[1] *Textbook of Psychology*, 1892, p. 464.

cept never varies; and between such unvarying terms the relations must be constant and express eternal verities."[1] And again, "We have concepts not only of qualities and relations, but of happenings and actions; and it might seem as if these could make the conceptual order active. But this would mean a false interpretation. The concepts are fixed, even though they designate parts which move in the flux; they do not act, even though they designate activities; and when we substitute them and their order, we substitute a scheme the intrinsically stationary nature of which is not altered by the fact that some of its terms symbolize changing originals."[2]

This passage opens a question which I have discussed elsewhere; the question of the relation between 'terms' or word symbols[3] and the 'concepts' or mental symbols which they denote. At present I hold the opinion that 'terms' must be regarded as relatively static and stable labels by which we denote the living and growing mental symbols or 'concepts' of which our knowledge is composed.

The early progenitors of historic man acquired the primitive elements of knowledge before they

[1] *Some Problems of Philosophy*, p. 53.
[2] *Ibid.*, pp. 81, 82.
[3] "Meaning and Error," *Journal of Philosophical Studies*, April, 1929, and Chapter iii of this book.

discovered language, and discovered language before they constructed logic; and to regard the mental symbols or ' concepts ' of which our knowledge is composed as being rigid and stable like the verbal symbols we use to denote them is to adopt a view under which a genetic theory of psychology becomes impossible, and logic becomes a rigid framework with which we try to embrace a reality which is changeful, elusive, and, by such means, unattainable.

A clue to the resolution of this impasse had previously been given by James himself in his *Textbook*. It runs thus: " In logic a concept is unalterable; but what are popularly called our ' conceptions of things ' alter by being used." [1] To follow this clue is to enquire: (1) What is the nature of the alterations which take place in ' our conceptions of things '? and (2) How are these ' conceptions of things ' related to ' logical concepts '? Thirty years' work on the subject enabled me to show that we may regard concepts

[1] Wm. James, *Textbook of Psychology*, 1891, p. 327.
A similar view has recently been put forward by Prof. McDougall in a paper on " The Confusion of the Concept,' '*Journ. of Philosophical Studies*, January, 1929. But it would seem that neither logic nor psychology can be considered as other than complementary if diverse categories of what we call ' knowledge ' and as such must conform to any coherent and accepted ' theory of knowledge.' If these views of James and McDougall should find themselves in conflict with such a theory it may well be doubted whether they could long maintain for themselves the atmosphere in which alone they could permanently flourish.

as living mental symbols subject to a process of organic growth—a growth in mass or bulk accompanied by increasing differentiation of structure. To see this and all the implications inherent in such a view is to be within reach of a comprehensive theory of knowledge which is congruous on the one hand with a genetic psychology, and, on the other, with ascertained phenomena of the neural basis of our minds, the cerebro-spinal nervous system. I have elsewhere [1] formulated such a theory of knowledge as being concerned with " acquiring, differentiating, correlating and integrating percepts and concepts," and I have shown how this formula has implicit in it all the various processes which we call ' mental ' and which are concerned with and comprise what we ordinarily call ' knowledge ' and what we ordinarily call ' thought.' In this book and in subsequent papers I reached the conclusion that the mental symbols or concepts of which our knowledge and thought are ultimately composed are subject to a process of growth much like that of the different organs and parts of the body, a growth in mass or bulk accompanied by differentiation both of structure and of function. If this be a valid contention its implications are very far-reaching and with ' knowledge ' and ' thought' resolved into these relatively simple elements and

[1] *Elements in Thought and Emotion.*

processes we are much nearer to a synthetic or synoptic view which will embrace ' thought-processes ' or ' mental processes ' on the one hand and neural processes on the other.

Any attempt to arrive at a synthetic view which will embrace a theory of knowledge in its relation to neural processes must take account of the conclusions of traditional psychology; and amongst these is the one which has been handed down to us in the term ' dispositions.'

It has been one of the radical mistakes of a too-traditional psychology to have effected something of a divorce between some of the larger aspects of mental life by means of its abstractions—' cognitive,' ' affective ' and ' conative ' dispositions. This has brought about a widespread conception that these aspects of consciousness can be treated apart from one another without regard to their mutual interpenetration and interaction. In the usage which has grown up as a result of this, what we call ' interest ' is in this arrangement of terms ' affective,' but every conceivable subject or object in which man either ever does or ever can possibly 'take an interest' is 'cognitive.' To stereotype a crude antithesis by these outworn psychological abstractions is to falsify the situation. The two aspects of consciousness interpenetrate one another and interact in every process of reflection and expression.

To realize fully this mutual interpenetration is to be freed from the thraldom of the sterile and unreal abstractions ' cognitive ' and ' affective,' and to be enabled to see the active participation of both these aspects of consciousness in our ordinary processes of perception and of thought.   The work of Bergson and Freud has gone far in the direction of loosening the tenure of this traditional usage, but the conclusions of the latter have, in the opinion of the writer, been vitiated by illogical inferences drawn largely from psychopathic cases —inferences which have tried alike the fidelity of many of his disciples and the gravity of many of his critics.

From the psychological standpoint here briefly outlined we approach the psychoneural problem with the concept as the ultimate constituent element of what have long been called our ' cognitive dispositions '; this concept being a living plastic mental symbol subject to a process of organic growth, its growth also being due to an affective factor which is constantly at work determining the selection of new sense data *from the perceptual flux, interpenetrating the conceptual contents of our minds, and integrating all these various and varying constituents into the slowly maturing dispositions which constitute our organized ' knowledge.'   The affective factor here involved has been variously termed ' libido,' ' love,' ' interest,' ' feeling,' ' desire,' ' liking,' etc.   I have elsewhere* [1] *considered and treated it in relation to the multitudinous conceptual contents of our minds, and outlined its part in fashioning the various ' emotions ' and ' sentiments.'*

' Dispositions ' have been defined by Stout as " the abiding after-effects left behind by prior experiences: they are inherited and acquired." [2] If this definition of ' dispositions ' be one which is generally accepted by psychologists we may regard the term as denoting the psychological aspect or expression of that part of the hypothetical psychoneural structures and processes which are called by Richard Semon ' engrammic systems ' [3] and from the neurological standpoint are termed by Head and Holmes ' neural schemata,' [4] but with which they have not yet been brought into due and necessary correlation. When this shall have been done it will become apparent that we shall be within reach of a synoptic view

[1] See chap. vi, on " The Conceptual and Emotional Complexes " in my *Elements in Thought and Emotion.*

[2] Stout's *Groundwork of Psychology,* p. 7.

[3] It is held by many that Semon's ' engrams ' have no neurological significance and should be dismissed with others of the somewhat uncouth terms in which he enshrined his psychological tenets. In *The Mneme* (p. 24) he defined the ' engram ' as " a permanent change wrought by a stimulus on any irritable living substance "; and in view of the fact that in *Mnemic Psychology* he continually used this term in immediate reference to ' sensations ' in human beings it seems to the writer difficult to deny it a neurological implication. For this reason he has come, rightly or wrongly, to regard it as a permissible synonym for Head's term ' neural schema,' or Morton Prince's ' neurogram.'

[4] Henry Head and Gordon Holmes, " Sensory Disturbances from Cerebral Lesions." *Brain,* vol. xxxiv.

embracing the formulated conclusions of psychologists on the one hand and neurologists on the other.

In the previous chapter[1] I had occasion to review some of the work of Richard Semon and of Head and Holmes, and was driven to the conclusions:

(1) That the 'engrams' or 'engrammic systems' of Semon were identical with the 'neural schemata' of Head and Holmes, these terms or phrases both denoting systems of neural paths between different areas of the brain—paths which had been developed and had become functional in the course of the ontogenic life history.

(2) That these 'engrams' or 'schemata' furnished the neural correlates of the multitudinous psychological elements which, when integrated into a more or less coherent aggregation of mental symbols or concepts constitute what we ordinarily call 'knowledge' and which in their interactions and ever-changing functional relations constitute what we ordinarily call 'thought-processes.'

(3) That a cursory consideration of the ordinary phenomena of 'memory,' 'reverie' and the different phases of what we call 'ratiocination' makes evident the need of a means of activating the

---

[1] " The Neural Substrata of Reflective Thought."

multitudinous 'engrams' or 'schemata' from some central source quite apart from any stimuli from the sense organs or receptors.

(4) That the central source of power to maintain a continuous stream of neural impulse, ever changing in the pattern of its flow through the multitudinous systems of ' engrams ' or ' schemata' is furnished by the thalami; and

(5) That the return paths from cortex to thalami—the cortico-thalamic paths—are means of maintaining a continuous circulation of neural impulse between the thalami and the cortex, thus keeping in an active state those 'engrams' or ' schemata ' which form the neural correlates of the mental symbols or concepts which may be employed in any particular phase of consciousness through which we may at any time be passing.

Here then is what must indeed at present be regarded only as a working hypothesis, but one which subsequent research may convert into an established theory—the hypothesis that the thalami which Head and Holmes regarded as the central seat of consciousness for the affective aspect of sensation, act also as central propagators of streams of neural impulse to all the ' engrammic systems ' or ' neural schemata ' which form the neural bases of our thought-processes, much as the heart propels the stream of blood through the whole vascular system.[1]   In so doing the thalami are concerned with activating the ' engrams ' or ' neural schemata ' which form the neural bases of the mental symbols or concepts.   In this way the thalami contribute the neural correlate of what from a psychological standpoint is the affective factor, participating in all our processes of perception and thought.   For in every act of perception there is a commingling and interaction of *a priori data* and *sense data*: the *a priori data* consisting of the conceptual contents of the mind and also of the affective factor which interpenetrates and activates them; and water does not run downhill more persistently than does the affective factor influence the selection of new *sense data* from the perceptual flux.   The *sense data* are from the neurological standpoint afferent neural impulses transmitted from the various receptor end-organs.

In a paper on " The Organic Growth of the Concept as one of the Factors in Intelligence [2] " I sketched in outline from the psychological point of view the growth during a period of two decades of my own concept of Sir Arthur Keith, showing to some extent the interaction of the so called

---

[1] This analogy seems justifiable as an illustration, although the streams of neural impulses must be held to be subject to an ever-changing direction among the multitudinous neural paths, and to be subject also to what we usually call ' volition,' while the stream of blood is not.

[2] *Brit. Journ. of Psychol.*, vol. xix, pt. i, July, 1928, and Chapter ii.

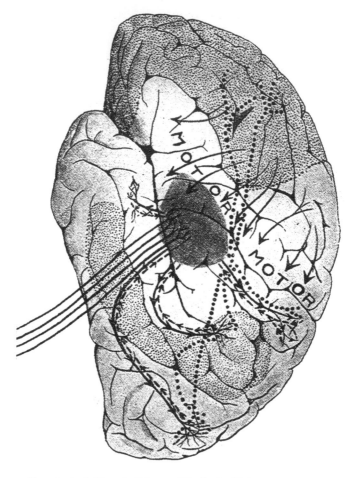

Hypothetical Neural Schema (Head & Holmes), Engrammic
System (Semon), or Neurogram (Morton Prince).

Thalamo-cortical and fronto-motor paths—continuous lines.
Cortico-thalamic paths—intermittent lines.
Association paths—dotted lines.

[face p. 109

'cognitive' and 'affective' factors in its various processes of growth, and how the interaction of this concept with others is due to the affective factor in consciousness. In the accompanying figures (pages 109 and 110) an attempt has been made to illustrate in bare essentials the 'engrammic system,' 'neural schema' or 'neurogram' which on the hypothesis here presented must be held to form in my own brain the concept's neurological substratum. If a 'disposition' be correctly defined as "the abiding after-effects left behind by prior experiences" the 'engrammic system' or 'neural schema' may be held to stand for its neurological embodiment. The thalami are seen in the diagrams in their approximate relations to the cortex. Adopting the view of Head and Holmes that the essential thalamic organs are the neurological seat of the affective aspects of sensation, the neural impulses which contribute to the slow development of this 'engrammic system' or 'neural schema' are held to come largely from the essential thalamic organs as well as from the exteroceptor end-organs. These impulses from the thalami are held to furnish also the neural correlate of the affective factor which is continually at work in our thought-processes and in every act of perception.

The diagrammatic 'engrammic system' or 'neural schema' here sketched may prove to be largely erroneous. This will turn much on the arrangement and distribution in the thalamic fan or radiation of the thalamo-cortical (thalamo-fugal) and cortico-thalamic (cortico-fugal) paths. Does the original path through, *e.g.*, the sensory visual area to the visual word area become in the course of development supplemented by paths direct from the thalami to the word area, and are such new circuits being gradually established and made functional in all parts of the brain during the entire course of our ontogenetic mental growth? The phylogeny of the parts concerned, when viewed in the light of Hughlings Jackson's doctrine of the evolution of the nervous system, would seem to justify the inference that such new circuits are continually being developed and being brought by facilitation into a condition of functional dominance, but we touch here on a speculative question which seems likely to elude our present methods of direct investigation.

Pen in hand, I may be writing to this person on some semi-recondite subject the consideration of which, as I write, necessitates my referring to some book for verification of a point on which I am doubtful. When my doubts are resolved my argument develops, largely by means of the activity of the cortical association areas which constitute the largest and phylogenetically the latest of man's neural structures for the harmonious and

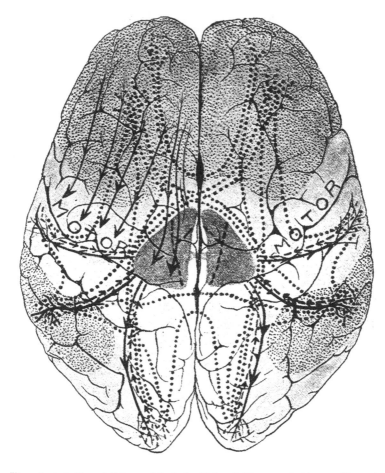

Hypothetical Neural Schema (Head & Holmes), Engrammic System (Semon),
or Neurogram (Morton Prince).

Thalamo-cortical and fronto-motor paths—continuous lines.
Cortico-thalamic paths—intermittent lines.
Association paths—dotted lines.

[face p. 110

balanced integration of a life-time's perceptual experience. If this be so, these structures may be regarded as contributing much to the neurological basis of what has long been called ' reason,' and the immediate juxtaposition of the frontal association areas to the cortical motor area facilitates, at once, the translation of what we call ' judgments' into written or spoken words, or other appropriate actions.

With these considerations in mind, the question arises: What are the psychological implications of the fact that one of the latest and most important of the ' association areas' in man has been developed in such intimate juxtaposition with the cortical motor areas, and, further, what is the bearing of this on the oddities of the doctrine which is called ' behaviourism '?

Fourteen years ago it was possible for Head to say: "Most observers start with the assumption that impulses originate in the peripheral end-organs and pass unaltered to the cortex, there to underlie that psychical state we call a sensation." [1] The validity of this statement is well shown in many of the diagrams which have been constructed to illustrate the grouping of the multitudinous paths to be found in the cortex. To contemplate these for a time is to be put in mind of a township with the streets and houses admirably fitted with an

[1] Sir Henry Head, *Studies in Neurology*, vol. ii, p. 601.

elaborate system of wiring for electric light, but which is supplied by cables from an adjoining place, the township having no central generating station of its own. As long as supplies from the outside continue all goes well, but when these are cut off, the township, being unable to generate current for itself, is left in entire darkness. In the hypothesis here presented the thalami are held to subserve four different but intimately co-ordinated functions, viz. those of acting as:

(1) The junctions and distributing stations for all sensory impulses (Head and Holmes).

(2) The central organs or seats of the affective aspects of sensation (Head and Holmes).

(3) The means of furnishing by their essential organs the affective factor which is an essential ingredient of every act of perception; and

(4) The means, by innumerable conditioned and unconditioned reflexes in their essential organs, of sending neural impulses to all parts of the cortex during our various processes of reflective and ir-reflective thought, when these are working spontaneously and entirely cut off from intruding perceptual interference.

The thalami may be said to have long figured as Cinderellas among the cerebral organs where they have been kept in the background and in a constant state of being repressed by inhibitory impulses passing along the cortico-thalamic paths. The hypothesis here presented brings them into the foreground of the picture and assigns to their activities a primary position not merely in the affective, but also in the cognitive processes. Co-operating with impulses from the exteroceptor end-organs to activate the multitudinous ' engrams ' or ' schemata ' which constitute the neural basis of the elements of what we call ' knowledge ' and what we call ' thought-processes,' they also maintain a continuity of neural impulses, ever changing in the direction of their flow—impulses which are able to activate the same ' engrams ' or ' schemata ' in those phases of the ' thought-processes ' which take place unmixed with the influence of new perceptual experience.

The monumental work which has been performed by Head and his collaborators in the study of the regrouping in the thalami of the sensory impulses from the lower physiological levels requires to be done with like discriminating exactitude and laborious pains at the higher sensory levels which are concerned with the impulses transmitted by those cranial nerves which make their contribution to what we call the ' special senses.' For any one who will devote a life-time to this study there will come a rich harvest; and the material for it lies ready to hand in Head's masterly studies of pathological and traumatic varieties of

H

Aphasia [1] and his insistence on the employment of Hughlings Jackson's method of approach to such cases by way of psychology. In such a study there lie implicit and will gradually be revealed the highly complex interactions between what we call the ' cognitive ' and what we call the ' affective ' aspects of consciousness. This will become more apparent from a prolonged study of the regrouping in the thalami, of impulses from the nerves of special sense and the relation of these regrouped impulses to the essential thalamic organs, viewing those organs in the light of Head's conclusion that they constitute the neurological basis of what we call the affective aspect of consciousness.

The great body of work done by Head and his collaborators, and by Richard Semon, the train of conceptions which, in the course of years, led to their matured views and are implicit in their phrases ' neural schemata ' and ' engrammic systems ' may be found in the long run to mark a turning point in the history of the investigation of the psycho-neural problem. They seem to turn our minds more into the direction of a functional consideration of the subject as distinguished from a mere anatomical localization of functional areas and glib generalities about ' incito-motor centres.' It has been largely through their

[1] Sir Henry Head, *Aphasia and Kindred Disorders of Speech.*

work that I was led to the position here outlined
which seems to give a unitary coherence to the
neurological processes of thalamo-cortical functioning. If the hypothesis here presented has in
it the elements or outline of a reliable theory,
men's minds will gradually be drawn that way;
but it must be interpreted in the light of all that
I have elsewhere written on the kindred subjects
of psychology and epistemology which are bound
up with it. It will be only by considering synoptically and finding an integration of all the aspects
of the problem that a reasonable solution of the
psychoneural workings of man's mind will in
the end be reached.[1]

The hypothesis here presented finds itself
launched into a neurological world imbued with
a view which has been growing into general ac-
ceptance for nearly two decades, and with which
it must at first seem, and even, perhaps, on further
consideration prove to be, in fundamental antag-
onism. This view is one in which the varied
complexities of observed phenomena in many

[1] Prof. Stopford (*loq.*) : " What about patients with destruction of
part or the whole of a thalamus ? "
    Sir Grafton Elliot Smith: "I would put the same query as Stopford."
The writer : " So would I."
    The answer to this query may conceivably come in another generation
as the result of prolonged and adequate clinical study of the progressive
ante-mortem changes of psychic states in such cases, and the subsequent
correlation of the results of this study with the findings of the post-
mortem examinations.

pathological cases find a summarized expression
of thalamic functioning in such phrases as 'cortical
control' and 'syndrome thalamique.' Implicit in
the view indicated by these phrases is the belief
that the cortex exercises a tonic control over
the functioning of the thalami by means of the
cortico-thalamic paths, and that when this influence or control is abolished by a sufficiently widespread derangement of these paths the thalami,
' released ' from ' cortical control,' are free to exert
their affective functions in various primitive and
disordered ways.   On so important a matter of
difference controversy may hinge for a generation,
and at the outset it may be well to delimit as far
as possible the precise point at issue.

It is agreed on all hands that amongst the multitudinous neural paths which connect and function
between the thalami and the cortex there are some
which transmit impulses from thalami to cortex
(thalamo-cortical, thalamo-fugal) and others which
transmit impulses from cortex to thalami (cortico-
thalamic, cortico-fugal).   The central point at
issue upon which the opposed views turn, is, what
functions do the impulses perform which pass
along the cortico-thalamic (cortico-fugal) paths?
The main facts are not in dispute; the question is
one of their interpretation; and here precisely is
the point where I desire to join issue.   Are these
impulses on the one hand, and as one view holds,

impulses inhibiting thalamic activity, or, on the other, are they concerned with keeping up, by means of conditioned and unconditioned reflexes in the essential thalamic organs, a varying continuity of neural impulse to activate the ' schemata ' or ' engrams ' which form the neural substrata of our thought-processes? This question is one upon which no compromise or agreement appears possible. It seems to admit of no gradations—of no less or more; and, if this be so, judgment must in the long run turn upon which view provides the better means of integrating a valid theory for explaining all the varied phenomena—psychological and neural—both in the ordinary processes of mental life and in the numerous kinds of psychopathic cases.

To treat this aspect of the subject with the adequacy demanded by the fundamental importance of the whole question would be to review it fully in the light of Hughlings Jackson's Croonian lectures on *The Evolution and Dissolution of the Nervous System*, and in the light also of the subsequent work of Head and others. To do this will involve the consideration of widespread data with a sufficiency of matter for more than one paper in the future. It will suffice for the present to indicate in outline the kind of view which seems implicit in the hypothesis presented here.

Let us turn to a crucial passage in Hughlings Jackson's [1] lectures:

" The doctrine of evolution implies the passage from the most organized to the least organized, or, in other terms, from the most general to the most special.   Roughly, we may say that there is a gradual 'adding on' of the more and more special, a continual adding on of new organizations.   But this 'adding on' is at the same time a 'keeping down.'   The higher nervous arrangements evolved out of the lower keep down those lower, just as a government evolved out of a nation controls as well as directs that nation.   If this be the process of evolution, then the reverse process of dissolution is not only a 'taking off' of the higher, but is at the very same time a 'letting go' of the lower.   If the governing body of this country were destroyed suddenly, we should have two causes for lamentation: (1) the loss of services of eminent men; and (2) the anarchy of the now uncontrolled people.   The loss of the governing body answers to the dissolution in our patient (the exhaustion of the highest two layers of his highest centres); the anarchy answers to the no longer controlled activity of the next lower level of evolution (third layer).

Another way of stating the general principle involved (Anstie's principle), is that the over-activity in epileptic mania and in the other cases mentioned, is not caused, but is permitted; on cutting across the pneumogastric, the heart is not caused to go faster, but is permitted to go faster.   In other words, the lower level of evolution is not 'goaded into activity,' but is 'let go.'   So we see that exhaustion of the highest nervous arrangements— two layers—answers to negative affection of consciousness; and this exhaustion being, at the same time, a removal of control from the next lower level of evolution—third—it springs into activity—is 'let go.' "

This passage was, of course, written before the question of the functioning of the thalami had

---

[1] *The Croonian Lectures*, reprinted from the *Brit. Med. Journ.* 1884, pp. 15, 16.

loomed into the foreground of the neurological vista; and the 'control' here referred to *is not the control of particular organs but of lower levels of neural organization.*

It is more than doubtful whether any known process of logic would permit the substitution of the term 'thalami' as an equivalent for the phrase 'next lower level of evolution' in the passage cited, or justify the added inference that the 'control' is due to inhibitory impulses passing along the cortico-thalamic paths.

Another analogy—from biology—may fitly be placed beside Hughlings Jackson's political one. About twenty-five years ago some of the upper branches of an oak-tree in my garden being dead, I cut through two large boughs into which the tree had forked near the top. This was soon followed by the bursting into activity of a number of buds which had long lain dormant but which now soon formed quite a forest of twigs. I watched them with interest and observed that in course of time two or three of these acquired functional dominance and ultimately grew into large branches while the others in the course of time became dwarfed and seemed to die away. The flow of sap being doubtless gradually adjusted to the branches which had become functionally dominant, the others gradually withered, leaving, no doubt, more dormant buds to repeat in case of need the performance of twenty-five years ago. I submit that this is a not inapt illustration of some phases of what takes place along some of the neural paths in the course of our ontogenetic mental growth. The exhaustion or incapacity from different causes of the higher levels of neural structure which have most recently attained functional status is the occasion of lower levels of earlier structural organization again resuming the functions which they had performed in an earlier stage of the ontogenetic process.

" For the use of language is based on integrated functions, standing higher in the neural hierarchy than motion or sensation, and, when it is disturbed, the clinical manifestations appear in terms of these complex psychical processes; they cannot be classed under any physiological categories, motor or sensory, nor even under such headings as visual and auditory." [1]

The girl in her teens who, when in a state of fever, talked volubly in Hindustani which she had learned in infancy and subsequently forgotten: the aphasic who could remember his own address but not that of his mother-in-law who lived with him: W. H. Hudson, who, in a period of mental exhaustion during a six weeks' illness, found memories of his forgotten past reviving so that he could write them down as he lay in bed: [2] the

[1] Sir Henry Head, *Aphasia and Kindred Disorders of Speech*, vol. i, p. 203.
[2] F. C. Bartlett, " Types of Imagination," *Journ. of Philosophical Studies*, vol. iii, pt. 9, p. 79.

recurrence in states of senility of long-forgotten memories of childhood—all cases such as these come within the range of the conditions here laid down by Hughlings Jackson. They are all explicable on the view that lower, earlier and partly disused levels of functioning come into activity again when higher and later ones fail. But there is no necessary implication here of any failure of presumed thalamic inhibition. Rather is it reasonable, in view of the phylogenetic history of the parts, to suppose that both thalami and cortex contribute together towards the formation of the different functional levels of neural structure which are successively formed during the onto-genetic life process, and that in the case of the failure of the higher levels the lower ones resume the more primitive functions which they performed in earlier periods of the individual life.

The considerations here adduced seem to show that an alternative view is possible to the one at present current of the function of the impulses transmitted by the cortico-thalamic paths, and that their real function may conceivably be to contribute their part towards a thalamo-cortical circulation of neural impulse.

CHAPTER VI

THE THALAMO-CORTICAL CIRCULATION OF NEURAL IMPULSE AND THE PSYCHO-NEUROSES

IN previous chapters I have set forth the hypothesis of a " Thalamo-cortical circulation of neural impulse," and shown its relation to the cognitive elements of what we usually call ' knowledge.' The thesis is that the continuity of the trains of what we call ' thought ' which are unceasingly passing through what we call our ' minds ' during the periods of what we call ' consciousness ' have their neural correlates in a continuity of neural impulse to and fro from thalami to cortex and from cortex to thalami along the multitudinous thalamo-cortico and cortico-thalamic paths in the thalamic fan or radiation. This hypothesis is congruous on the one hand with the conclusion at which Head and his collaborators laboriously arrived, that the thalami constitute the neurological centres for the affective aspects of sensation, and on the other hand with Alexander's conclusion that mental process must be identified with neural process.[1]

The acid test to which this hypothesis must in

---

[1] " We are forced, therefore, to go beyond the mere correlation of the mental with these neural processes and to identify them " (*Space, Time and Deity*, by Prof. S. Alexander, ii, 5).

future be submitted and from which it must
emerge, will, perhaps, be found in an answer to
the question—Does it help to throw light upon
and to explain those phenomena of aberrant
mental functioning which are usually grouped
under the term ' Psycho-neuroses '?

It is a first necessity in any attempt to answer
this question to perceive clearly the essential neurological implications of the hypothesis itself, and
these, as at present conceived in the ' mind ' of
the writer, are briefly as follows.

The various parts of the cortex we know to be
multitudinously interconnected by association
fibres and also by the cortical association areas;
but it is, too, a necessary implication of the hypothesis of a thalamo-cortical circulation of neural
impulse to suppose that the various thalamo-
cortical and cortico-thalamic tracts of fibres shall
also be functionally connected with one another
by inter-connexion cells in the deeper parts of
the *thalami*: that what we know as *cortical* association areas shall be acknowledged to have a counterpart also in the thalami, and it will be for neurologists to say whether these hypothetical thalamic
association areas lie in and constitute a chief part
of what Head has called " the essential thalamic
organs." If this be so the essential thalamic
organs must come to be regarded as neurological
regions performing functions for the *affective*

aspects of mind somewhat similar to those fulfilled by the cortical association areas in its *cognitive* aspects, and also in the more complex processes of transmuting intermingled cognitive and affective activities into their appropriate motor activities. In this view, the essential thalamic organs, functioning in close inter-relationship with the cortical functional areas, furnish the neurological correlates of what from a psychological point of view are the affective factors to be detected in every process of perception and of thought.[1]

We have then on this hypothesis four distinct kinds of intercommunication between the various parts of the entire system of thalamo-cortical functional areas:

(1) The cortical intercommunication tracts and association fibres connecting different functional areas in the cortex.

(2) The traditional cortical association areas of the anatomical textbooks. (Frontal and parieto-temporal.)

(3) The thalamo-cortical and cortico-thalamic paths.

[1] " Until recently, the part played by this organ (the thalamus) in sensation was unknown. But we now recognize that it is the seat of those physiological processes which underlie crude sensations of contact, pain, heat and cold, together with the feeling-tone they evoke. The essential organ of the optic thalamus is the centre for the effective aspect of sensation, whilst discrimination and spacial projection are the product of cortical activity " (*Studies in Neurology*, by Sir Henry Head, ii, p. 642).

(4) The essential thalamic órgans (Head) functioning as thalamic association areas.

All these are here regarded as integral parts of a whole, and as furnishing, with the multitudinous systems of neurones which they bring into functional relationship, a large part of the entire neural mechanism forming the vehicle of our various cognitive and affective processes and the means of transmuting these processes into the innumerable and diverse motor activities which enter into and form so large a part of the volitional and habitual occupations of our daily lives.

But even when all this shall have been amplified in due proportion and set out in full volume only one-half of the entire story will have been told, unless and until full expression shall also have been given to the interactions of the autonomic with the cerebro-spinal nervous system, and the effects which are continually being produced by the influence of these two systems on one another.

Phylogenetically the thalami mostly belong to an older part of the brain than the neopallium—a part which was dominant in the lower vertebrates and from which the neopallium was developed much later. To the thalami come all the afferent nerves of the cerebro-spinal nervous system and, mingled with the fibres from the spinal cord, are the various contributions from the different parts of the sympathetic and parasympathetic systems. In these organs the sympathetic and parasympathetic systems are brought into intimate, if indirect,[1] relations with the various parts of the cortex, and through the intercommunications thus established the cortex can influence the various systems of involuntary muscles and also the secretions of the ductless glands.

If this be a valid contention it would seem that the thalami may be assigned a functional rôle congruous with their central anatomical positions in the nervous system. The thesis here presented seems to require that they be functionally regarded as organs contributing largely to what Sherrington has termed " the integrative action of the nervous system."

In this view of thalamo-cortical relations it seems not improbable that psychology may find a clue to the solution of some of its difficulties and be led to a unification of the various conflicting views which are at present manifest within its ambit,[2] and through this

[1] At present we are without assured anatomical knowledge as to the intercommunication between the sympathetic and cerebro-spinal systems, but Professor Stopford tells me that evidence is accumulating in support of the view that efferent sympathetic paths arise from nuclei in the subthalamic region.

[2] Prof. C. S. Myers in his recent Presidential Address, Section Psychology, Brit. Assoc., London, 1931, says : " More than thirty years' experience has convinced me that a thorough familiarity with the practice and theory of the psycho-physical methods is essential for reliable systematic psychological investigations of any kind. It is largely to the uncontrolled genius of psychologically untrained experts in other fields that we owe the exaggerated importance which has been variously attached of late to conditional reflexes, sex, inferiority, behaviour, mental tests, correlations, etc., in psychology. Thus have often arisen the various schools of modern psychology, characterized by the same narrow bigotry as is to be found among contending religious

view may ultimately come the fundamental psychological law or theory which shall embrace, harmonize and integrate the various diversities of 'introspective,' 'faculty,' 'psycho-analytic,' 'hormic,' and 'behaviourist' psychology—a law or theory which will embrace all our cognitive and affective states of consciousness in relation to the neutral states by which they are conditioned.

The late W. H. R. Rivers at the beginning of his book, *Instinct and the Unconscious,* stated that " one of the chief aims of this book is to discover the nature and biological significance of the mechanism of suppression " (p. 18). At the end of his discussion of the subject he reached only the conclusion which he expressed in the phrase: " I regard suppression as an instinctive process " (p. 126), and of the neural processes by which suppression comes into being he could make no statement at all.

But with the above conception in our minds the imagination can almost riot in various neural possibilities by which, through a reconditioning of pre-established reflexes, this condition of suppression can come about. Accepting the conclusions of Head and his collaborators that the

sects, each school almost worshipping its founder, each contributing something of truth and value, but each refusing to recognize truth and value in its rivals, and blind to other important conceptions than its own and to other important problems the investigation of which is essential for the progress of psychological science."

thalami are the seats of the affective aspects of sensation and the cortex that of spacial projection and discrimination while serving also as "the storehouse of past impressions,"[1] and remembering also that the nerve fibres entering the thalami, whether from the fillet or from the cortex, terminate in arborizations among the neurones of those organs, a change of conditioning of the pre-established reflexes, however brought about, may so change the paths of incoming sensory impulses as to divert them from their accustomed "neural schemata" (Head) in the cortex which constitute the neural substrata of the cognitive part of this past experience. Thus diverted from their accustomed paths to the cortex these impulses may then, in their aberrant courses in the thalami, affect the sympathetic and parasympathetic systems, producing those familiar symptoms of deranged organic processes which are characteristic of some of the psycho-neuroses, and which Pavlov produced experimentally in some of his dogs.

A case from McDougall's *Abnormal Psychology* illustrates this admirably:

Case 17, p. 266.

"A case of repressed memory. Neurasthenia with great emaciation. After a holiday was restored to health. Then repeated train journeys to business produced a serious relapse. Exploration in hypnosis disclosed suspected amnesia of a dis-

[1] *Studies in Neurology*, by Sir Henry Head, ii. p. 607.

tressing night journey in motor ambulance with several wounded soldiers. In the waking state he had been unable to recollect this journey. From the time of recovering his memory he made rapid recovery to normal health."

It is interesting to consider this case in immediate relationship to the hypothesis under consideration —a hypothesis which is quite largely the outcome of the laborious and monumental studies of Head and his collaborators. For this purpose it was necessary to select a case in which the disability was, so far as can be ascertained, a merely functional disorder and *not* one of pathological origin and significance such as might in some cases be disclosed by an abnormal post-mortem condition: *not* the result of some tumour or inflammatory process, but a condition which was apparently the outcome of a mental shock or trauma, resulting in a functional derangement amenable to treatment of the kind which was in this case actually applied; or treatment of the kind which Bernard Hart has so aptly denoted by the term " affective therapeutics."[1] Such cases are numerous and will occur in numbers to those who are concerned in the treatment of such neuroses.

McDougall's comment on the above case is as follows:

" In this case it would seem that the distressing memory was successfully repressed, until the travelling by railway stirred it

[1] Goulstonian Lectures, *The Psycho-neuroses*, 2nd edition, 1929, p. 151.

I

to greater activity; when, though there was no conscious recol-
lection, the distressful emotions affected the patient's consciousness in an obscure fashion and disturbed his organic functions.
The case thus illustrates what seems to be a general rule, namely,
that the affect of a complex can disturb visceral functions and
make itself felt as a mood, while the cognitive content remains
outside consciousness."

If the hypothesis here presented be valid it
seems to afford an explanation in terms of neurology of the way in which this complex condition
of combined amnesia and disturbed organic function may be brought about. If Head's conclusion
be valid that the cortex functions as the storehouse
of past impressions and experience, it would seem
that any influences which interrupt an accustomed
flow of neural impulse to the cortical regions
which formed the neural substrata of any particular past experience would *ipso facto* produce an
amnesia of that particular experience. If, on the
other hand, the thalami are the central organs
where the cerebro-spinal and autonomic systems
are brought most intimately into functional relationship, it is precisely in these organs that the
interruption of accustomed paths to the cortex
might cause a diversion of neural impulses to those
efferent fibres of the spinal cord which influence
the sympathetic system and so produce that disturbance of organic function which, with the amnesia, was so marked a feature of the case cited
above. The interruption of impulses through one

set of reflexes might thus result in the twofold disability, being primarily the actual immediate cause of the amnesia, and secondarily that of the disturbed organic function owing to the diversion of neural impulses to the sympathetic. The restoration of the lost memory would on this hypothesis imply that the neural impulses were once again taking their normal courses to the cortex with a cessation of their diversion to those tracts of the sympathetic where they acted to the detriment of the visceral functions.

This view seems to the writer entirely congruous with Janet's teaching " that dissociation is due to lack of mental synthesis subsequent upon a lowering of nervous tension" [1]; and it may be that we shall have to cease regarding many such cases as due to ' repression ' resulting from ' mental conflict.'

[1] " Psychotherapeutics and Psychopathology," by T. W. Mitchell. *Brit. Med. Journ.*, September 23, 1922.

EPILOGUE

It now remains for us to try and give a concrete illustration of the working of some of these neural processes as they are manifested in the social intercourse of everyday life. A scene from Miss Constance Holme's novel *The Lonely Plough* provides, in the description of the Agricultural Show in Chapter XIII, a suitable as well as humorous situation for this purpose. Beside the description we have placed in parallel columns notes of the accompanying neural processes as set forth in this book.

Let us begin with a thumb-nail sketch of some of the Dramatis Personæ. This may be helpful to those who are not acquainted with the book.

Bluecaster.—Local Lord and property owner. A young but sympathetic landlord.

Lancelot Lancaster.—Bluecaster's agent, aged thirty-seven. An acute, sound man of the land, with a clear-sighted view of terms and tenants, with " sympathy and idealism shrouded like sin."

Helwise.—Lancaster's aunt and housekeeper. A chattering piece of inconsequence who talked " like a string of telephone wires touching in a wind." " She had the aimless velocity of a trundled hoop, and accomplished about as much."

Hamer Shaw.—A business man who had retired a year previously from living luxuriously on the outskirts of a Lanca-

shire town. A large-hearted man who " would sooner have
shut his door on a Royal honour than on an old acquaintance."

DANDY SHAW.—Hamer Shaw's daughter, aged twenty-four.
A charming and well-educated member of society.

HARRIET KNEWSTUBB.—Occupant of Wild Duck Hall and
farm which she managed herself with the aid of a good
man. There was not much about farming which she did
not know.

FAWCETT KNEWSTUBB.—Harriet's father. " He was very
horsy, very check, utterly selfish and a really strong con-
noisseur in language and whisky. Harriet kept him and
his hunters, called him ' Stubbs! ' in the voice of a sergeant,
and wished him dead in a bitter heart."

" Hamer and his daughter motored to Bluecaster Show along
a road swarming with enthusiasts who had no notion of making
room for anybody. Dandy felt more of an outsider than ever
in the crowded field, with its jumping and cattle rings, its tents,
its long lines of wooden stands. She saw many faces she had
come to know, but few held return signs of recognition. The
usual people were busy greeting each other, very contented,
very much at home. They were there because they had always
been there since the time they could first sit on a stand without
falling through. After the greetings they buried their heads in
their catalogues and slouched along from pen to pen, walking
blindly into everybody else, and offering information to the empty
air. Anxious to do the thing thoroughly, Dandy and Hamer
bought catalogues and slouched, too. By this means they were
successful in running into Harriet, leaning up against something
extremely solid with four legs and a horn or two, gloating over
the blue-ribboned card opposite. When Hamer's catalogue
knocked her hat sideways, she merely remarked, ' How's that
for beef? ' and continued to gloat. It was a minute or two
before they could call her back to earth, but as soon as she
realized their existence she left off gloating, and trotted them
round the field in a terrific whirl of instruction, leading them at
last, somewhat stunned, to a seat on the grandstand.

The day was brilliant, but Harriet, defended against all odds by Donegal, Burberry and K., with a huge carriage-umbrella tucked under her arm, insisted stoutly that you never could tell. It always rained at Bluecaster Show—everybody knew that—and it would rain to-day; this in a tone indicating that it jolly well better had.   Dandy, dressed with the delicacy of a Blue Wyandotte, felt abashed until she discovered that Harriet was practically alone in her gloomily-barometric choice of attire.

Ringed in its green cup brimmed by blue hills, the scene had its own untheatrical charm, but its thrills were mild and long in arriving.   Business went forward with little regard to spectators, and, after a tedious half-hour, during which four horses, eight cows and twelve sheep stared solemnly at the crowd, while the whole Committee got down into the ring and wrangled about them, Dandy found her thoughts straying to the social ethics of the meeting.

There was a rail dividing the stand, cleaving the two-shilling section from the half-crown.   This puzzled her, as the planks on either side were equally hard.   Harriet's explanation that you got sixpenny-worth more water-jump scarcely seemed to go deep enough.   The grinders were half-crowners, she noticed, glued as a rule to the side of some local celebrity, such as the Member, or the High Sheriff, or the President ; but the leeches only ran to two shillings—with the exception of Helwise, who was inviting Bluecaster to come and see how badly they wanted a new bath at Crabtree, when she wasn't issuing orders to Lanty in the ring.

This illustrates the generalized statement in the Prologue that for the average man the power of perception in any particular scene is contingent on the conceptual knowledge in his cognitive dispositions at the time.

Apart from his aunt, Lancaster was having the usual harried time of an authority on these occasions.   When he wasn't helping or looking for the judge, he was calling competitors or catching stray sheep, artfully eluding business demands from button-holing tenants, or rescuing the usual veterans of the ring who stand so trustingly behind the hurdles.   He knew every-

Harriet and Lancaster had been made familiar by many repetitions year after year with details of this annual event, but to Hamer and Dandy, new to it all, the detailed interpretation was impossible. In Harriet and Lancaster the cortex was acting as the 'storehouse of past impressions' (Sir Henry Head) and the neural schemata previously formed were reacting to the present stimulus in terms of past experience, comparing present experience with past happenings, this being contingent on the intimate functioning of the whole series of neural schemata which had resulted from the aggregated past experience.

Affective processes involving in the circuit of neural impulse the hypothalamus, thalamus and cortex.

body, it seemed, just as Helwise, talking baths, knew everybody, and Harriet, flourishing her clumsy gamp. To Dandy names passing from mouth to mouth were no more than empty sound. The fact that Seaman was jumping did not fill her with anticipation, nor could the recent death of a well-known horseman move her to a sense of loss. She began to be rather bored by the unhurrying succession of events, and checked herself guiltily in a yawn. The judge of the moment was having a real day out with a fine hunter-class, and had to be practically dragged off each horse in turn. Hamer was drinking in Harriet's observations like an eager child, but he was as new to it all as his daughter.

Even the old hands were getting a little weary, and found time to turn a speculative eye upon the strangers— the cheery, handsome man and the slim, well-groomed girl; and the legend went round in ascending chromatics of incredulity. Some knew Hamer by accident, so to speak: 'Behaved very decently over that Abbey Corner smash, don't you know! Sporting and all that—gave a thumping big subscription to to-day's business,' etc. etc., and wondered vaguely whether he might not be worth cultivation. The women with sons looked at Dandy and said that anybody married anybody nowadays, and that even Kitchen Tea might be made positively chic if the butter were spread thick enough. The women with daughters only were not interested.

Dandy had ceased to be self-conscious, however. She was watching Lancaster at work with the same dreary chill of separation that she had experienced in the Lane. This was his life, the interchange of business and friendship to which she was an absolute stranger. Harriet was perfectly at ease in it, grumbling, grunting, cracking a joke with a passing farmer or summing up a prize-winner in a pithy sentence — at ease and happy.

' Dull enough to you, I expect,' she observed, detecting Dandy's secret yawn. 'We're brought up to it, of course. Besides, it's my trade. Rotten show, though! Rotten judging! Fool of a crowd. But all the same I couldn't stop away, any more than Lanty Lancaster. I've grown to it, you see. When I was a kid it was my big blow-out of the year, and I've still got the same feeling for it, like Christmas Day and all that piffle. It isn't the thing itself—it gets slacker and rottener every year, as I'm always telling them, especially Lanty Lancaster—it's what it stands for, and all the years behind it. If ever I want to purr, it's when I'm sitting on this shaky old stand, watching a flat-footed imitation of a horse going slap for the water. But you must be about fed up on it, I

A statement of the power of habit and tradition in one individual, and its hold on the affective interest of whole cortical dispositions.

suppose! It's as slow as Noah's Ark, and, besides, it always rains.' She slipped the catch of the gamp to see if it worked, and shot a glance at the sun which should have sent it slinking over the horizon like a dog shouted to kennel. 'We're getting through to the jumping, though. You'll find that a bit more enlivening. Stubbs is turning out—did I tell you? He's got a mount that can jump about as much as a hedgehog, but he thinks he's going to win all right. It's no use my jawing; he won't take anything from me. I hope he'll behave decently, that's all, and not get slanging the judges. Trust Stubbs to have been where the sun is shining, even though it always rains!'

The band behind the stand broke into a dirge which proved to be 'The Girl in the Taxi,' and to this suitable motif the leapers sidled into the ring for their primary reconnaissance. There was something of the dignity of ritual in their solemn progression from fence to fence, in the measuring thrust of the intelligent heads through the furze. Dandy had her first thrill in spite of the accompaniment. She wanted to beat a little drum in the wake of the processional hoofs.

Harriet knew the riders, gentleman, groom, or horse-dealer, just as she knew the mounts—from the hunter, that did a little gentle following of hounds by the aid of gates, to the pro-

An anticipation, from past experience stored in the cortex, of what might and did happen later in the day.

Further recapitulation of past experience drawn from the storehouse of the cortex and stimulated into activity

by present phenomena of a similar kind.

fessional ' leppers ' that never see open country, but spend their time winning prizes at a round of shows, and jump more with their brains than with any other section of their queer-shaped carcasses. She dragged out a pencil like a poker, and settled down to work.

Continued recapitulation of past experience excited by present surroundings.

' That's Captain Pole-Pole on Griselda, the little grey. Rushes everything that she doesn't take stick at, and a brute to hold, by the look of her. The big roarer waving its wild tail and doing an imitation of a charging squadron belongs to Bluecaster. Lanty has her out for the fun of the thing. They call her something idiotic—oh yes— Flossie! She can jump quite a bit— —Heavens knows how—though you can feel the stand shake. There's a groom up—plays the triangle in my village orchestra. The thing called Chipmunk, looking as though it was made of knitting-needles, belongs to the Ritson Bros. One's riding, and the other runs in and throws things if Chippie starts frivolling. There's the winner—the little brown like an oak-box with head and legs. You'd think he hadn't the reach for a grass-plot rail, but he's there, every time. Watch his eyes and his good-tempered ears! He's as pleased as punch all along, and as dead in earnest as a city man sprinting for his train. Yes, he'll win right enough! Why? Because he jumps with his head. You can see him stop to think just before he takes off, and he doesn't give the fence an inch more than is wanted. This is his living—he comes from Saddleback way—and little Seaman doesn't mean to waste himself playing round. Stubbs must be cracked to think he can beat him! The rough-looking black with the rope-reins has been taught to behave like a mad circus and an Ulster riot combined. Its owner is a blacksmith in his spare time, and nobody else can stick on its back. It's clever, too, but it's apt to get carried away by its play-acting and make mistakes. Flyer goes to sleep and leaves his heels behind him, and Grace tries to do the tight-rope act on the pole with all four feet at once. That's Stubbs on his beetle-crusher—Lapwing, he calls it! He doesn't look any too genial, does he? We had a row before starting, about rotifers, if you know what those are—some sort of a measly swimming microbe or rotten reptile of that kind. It's the only thing he cares a rap about except horses and the inside of a glass, and he was ramping mad because some of the beastly things had got thrown away. I hope Lanty is somewhere about.'

A preliminary reference to one of Stubbs' hobbies which was used to good purpose by Hamer later in the day.

Stubbs was immense—very check, very baggy, and very red in the face. His side-whiskers bristled aggressively, and there was a vicious gleam in his eye. He was riding a boring chestnut with weak quarters and the action of a schoolboy in clogs. Harriet dug the

person in front of her with the gamp
by way of relieving her feelings.
Hamer and Dandy tried to think of
things to say, but she cut them short.

' Oh, it won't be the first time he's
made fools of us both in public! I
can't help feeling a bit grubbed, but I
suppose I can stick it out. Anyhow,
I've got to stop and see him through.
Save them hunting me up if he goes
and breaks his neck.'

She thrust her hands in her pockets
and scowled. Lapwing had already
collided with the brown, and Stubbs,
ripe for fight, was beginning to ex-
plode. The quiet little boy on Seaman
stared in astonishment, until Lancaster, coming up, laid a palm on Lapwing's poking nose and drew him out
of range. He had some tale ready,
peculiarly adapted to Stubbs' appreciation, and Harriet caught her father's
guffaw as he rode to his side. She
sighed sharply—with relief, Dandy
judged—and addressed herself to shouting ' Good lad! ' or ' Good lass! ' with
supreme and delightful unconscious-
ness of self.

The sleepy Flyer led off, and left
everything in ruins behind him, after
which there was a lengthy pause, while
rails and bricks were replaced and
furze-tops refixed. Griselda gave a
charming illustration of the so-called
feminine temperament, refusing to look
at any jump until forced upon it, and
then flying it with a complete trust in

Providence and an absolute disregard
of economy. After these, the performance of the Bluecaster warrior
ranked high, in spite of the roaring
and waving accompaniment, and a
suggestion of clanking chains as she
rocked past. Carrying her proud head
at the noble angle affected by some
ladies much engaged in good works,
she yet contrived, by dint of squinting
down her nose at the last moment, to
view a jump in time to clear it, and
thundered on to the next in an atmosphere of escaped earthquakes.   In
spite of her size and weight, she
tackled the trap quite neatly, and
roared down the field to the water.
Here she was superb! On the wings
of sound she came, gathered herself
into a mighty bunch, plunged and was
over, leaving mingled impressions of
trumpets, bazaar bunting and a motor
exhaust.

Chipmunk did quite a good round,
thanks to a continuous shower of hats,
sticks, and ear-splitting yells, but
Grace's tight-rope effects were un-
successful except with the pole, on
which she managed to do quite a deli-
cate little bit of work.

Little Seaman had only one manner-
ism, a circular trot like the weaving
of a spell that seemed to wind him up
for the first hurdle. Dandy's heart
went out to the sensible, eager, square
little horse with the box-legs.   He
might have been a machine measured

to each length and lift, so obviously did he spare unnecessary effort, had it not been for clear evidence of mind behind, of humanly patient intelligence and endeavour. At the water, his customary check drew a groan of disappointment, changing to applause as it was seen that he was safely across. Certain ladies were so ear-piercingly enraptured that he had to drop on his knees and bow his little box-head before trotting soberly back to his place.

And, at last—Stubbs.

It was perfectly clear that Nature had never intended Lapwing to ' lep '; clearer still that Lapwing was entirely of Nature's opinion. He was born tired; his foolish head had a weary droop; his heavy hoofs were in curious contrast with his weedy frame. What he could not walk through, he sat on behind. When driven to rise, he hit the swing-gate with such force that he nearly looped the loop along with it. He bundled into the trap like a sack of old clothes, utterly abolished the stone wall, and plumped slick into the water, where he stayed determinedly, in spite of the volcanic eruption in the saddle. Lancaster removed the pair once more, this time with difficulty. Harriet flushed a little under the joy of the crowd, but she said nothing, only gave the same sharp little sigh as she watched the retreating figures and the soothing hand on the check knee.

A neural circuit involving hypothalamus, thalamus and cortex.

The second round brought its own disasters. Flyer had finally gone to sleep for the afternoon, and was withdrawn. Chipmunk missed the gate, owing to there being no hat handy. Only Seaman steadily kept his form—and Stubbs.

Lapwing came out as if he were going to be hanged. At the first hurdle he manifested pained surprise, stopped dead and began to nibble the furze. Blows and curses brought him to the straw-bound pole, where he again paused to munch. The gate being uneatable, however, he cleared it, pecking heavily, broke the trap into matchwood, and jammed his rider's knee against the wall. Then, evincing a sudden passion for the water, tore up to it con amore, only to swerve aside at the wing, leaving Stubbs to go on in the main direction; and as splash, roar and oath ascended to heaven, returned to his nibbling.

A tornado of emotional outburst involving hypothalamus, thalamus and cortex and issuing in the automatized mechanisms of certain speech habits. The persistence of Stubbs in his continued and repeated round of habitual word formulae affords an excellent example of the working of the thalamo-cortical circulation of neural impulse described in Chapter V, in which the hypothalamus also participates. This was kept up till it was

The Committee appeared on the spot like mushrooms. Stubbs was fished out, set right end up, condoled with, and, being close in front of the grandstand, requested to hush. But Stubbs did not hush, had no intention of hushing. Stamping and shouting, he informed them what he thought of shows in general and this show in particular. Then he was requested to leave, but he wouldn't do that, either, and by way of reply ran a coil of lurid language round every member

diverted by Hamer's adroit appeal to the stabilized series of neural schemata concerned with another permanent affective interest.

of the Association. Men climbed down from the stands and joined the happy party, until presently it seemed as if the whole Agricultural Society was helping in the suppression and ejection of Stubbs.

Harriet, white to the lips, observed ' Rotter! Low-down rotter! ' between her teeth and got to her feet; but when she would have made her way down, Hamer caught her by the arm.

' This isn't your job, my girl! ' he said, cheerfully, pressing her back into her seat. ' You stick to Dandy there, and grit your teeth a minute longer. I'll have things straightened out in two twos.'

He dropped into the ring with extraordinary lightness, while his daughter slipped a hand round Harriet's unreceptive elbow by way of conveying sympathy and keeping her quiet at the same time. Helwise fussed down to them, dropping things and repeating the bath-theme ad lib. The people near began to discuss hats and servants with feverish politeness, bringing a faint smile even to the victim's rigid lips. The Member stood up and tried to see something at the back of the stand that wasn't there, and of course all the grinders followed his example.

Hamer broke a path through the crush with his own pleasant directness of purpose. Everybody was trying to make Stubbs behave, and nobody was succeeding: neither Bluecaster, tongue-tied and ashamed, nor Lancaster, soothing and propelling, nor the High Sheriff, the Chief Constable, the Judges, the Secretary and Treasurer, the Referee in All Classes, nor the Police. It was a case of carrying Stubbs off bodily, and nobody liked to do it, for, in spite of language and check and abominable conduct, he was yet One of Us, and moreover his daughter watched from the stand. To them came Hamer the Outsider.

Hamer's appeal to the neural schemata of another permanent interest. Once made it is kept up by a slightly varied stimulus until Stubbs has been manœuvred into the car and driven off the field.

'Sir,' he observed to Stubbs, with the simple grace of touch that gave his every action charm, 'I understand you to be an authority upon Rotifera. I should like your advice upon the mounting of certain specimens of Bdelloidaceae that I have just obtained!'

Stubbs broke off half-way in a stream of adjectives beginning with the second and fourth letters of the alphabet, and stared; and everybody round, after a momentary impression that Hamer was drunk, too, wagged their heads and repeated 'Bdelloidaceae!' in a loud chorus, as if it were some kind of charm, until Stubbs himself began to say any bits of it that came foremost, without in the least meaning to.

'I have also some fine samples of Pedalionidae,' Hamer continued in

K

his comforting tones, motioning Lancaster to call up his car as he engineered the offender towards the rope. ' A remarkable species—most remarkable!—but perfectly familiar to you, I've no doubt. The Flosculariaceae, too, not to speak of the Philodinaceae —here we are, and mind the step! '

Stubbs made one last attempt to get up steam, but was throttled with a fresh animalcule, hustled into the car and driven off. Lanty came back to the girls.

' I'm to drive you home, if you'll allow me,' he said to Dandy; and ' Can I find your bicycle? ' to Harriet. ' The third round will be through in a few minutes, but I'll hand my job over to somebody, and we'll clear off at once, if you like. Your man has the horse, so he's all right. You've done well, to-day, haven't you ? How many firsts did you get ? You and Wild Duck are bad to beat! '

Harriet grunted, but her face relaxed. It hardened again, however, as she stood up and took a last defiant look round before walking off the field. She cycled home behind the dogcart, counting the times Lancaster's eyes were turned to Dandy's face. She was a trifle cheered when it began to rain heavily, and she was able to hand over the carriage-umbrella with an air of patronage, and splash along bravely in Burberry and K., but in spite of the ' firsts,' in spite of having been proved infallible, her cup of bitterness, that day, was full.

Helwise chattered all the way as blithely as if erring fathers and shamed daughters did not exist. Bluecaster, it seemed, had promised the bath.

'He was quite agreeable about it, Lancelot—porcelain on legs, nickel-plated hot and cold, you know! I really hadn't to hint more than twice! That led on, of course, to the Perils to Plumbers—my dear boy, how often have I told you that I never ask! He's sending the cheque to-night. You don't think, Miss Shaw, that your charming father——? Really, Lancelot, you needn't bite my head off! You're not a bit grateful about the bath, and I don't agree with you that the old one was all right. I knew I should get a present to-day, because I put on my skirt wrong side out. That always means luck! It was rather awkward, because the wrong side of the stuff doesn't go with the coat, and the picoted seams looked rather queer—I saw people staring, on the stand—but I'm glad I stuck to it! If I'd changed, I shouldn't have got the bath.'

Dandy listened vaguely to the chattering voice, thinking of her father, happily mounted on his favourite hobby. He would love looking after Stubbs, and they would spend the evening forming plans for his

Alternations of inconsequent thought and speech kept up by circuits of neural impulse between hypothalamus, thalamus and cortex.

Interactions of hypothalamus, thalamus and cortex which caused a mental absorption in which Helwise was entirely forgotten.

regeneration. She had a touch of tenderness for the impossible Stubbs; he had unintentionally given her this blissful ride in the rain. When Helwise stopped for a second, she listened to the hoofs and to Lanty's little clicks and calls of encouragement. She had heard him define horse-travelling as 'company and music.' She remembered it now, and had music in her heart to match. And so, in hearing it, forgot to listen to Helwise altogether.

.   .   .   .   .

And for a whole week the County talked of Hamer, and went about prating of Bdelloidaceae as if they bred them, and looked up rotiferous information on the quiet, in order to confound each other's ignorance. The wives called at Watters and filled the card-tray, and the postman staggered under letters of invitation. Hamer became known as 'sound,' 'useful,' 'a man at a pinch,' 'a dashed good sort all round, don't you know!' and every club in the district fought to own him. He was quite pleased about it all, and never guessed that his impulsive piece of 'tramming' had worked the transformation. Somebody in a hole needing pulling out was all that Hamer wanted to make him happy, and he was seldom out of a job. He welcomed the new friends as he had welcomed the grinders and leeches, and opened to them his heart and his pocket.

That was how Hamer became ' county '."

BIBLIOGRAPHY

ALEXANDER (S.). *Space, Time and Deity.* (Gifford Lectures at Glasgow, 1916–1918.) 2 vols. London, 1920.

—— "The Artistry of Truth." *Hibbert J.*, Jan. 1925.

BARTLETT (F. C.). "Types of Imagination." *J. Philosoph. Stud.*, iii, pt. 9, p. 79.

BERGSON (H.). *An Introduction to Metaphysics.* Transl. by T. E. Hulme. London, 1913.

BIANCHI (L.). *The Mechanism of the Brain and the Function of the Frontal Lobes.* Transl. by J. H. Macdonald. Edinburgh, 1922.

BOLTON (J. S.). *The Brain in Health and Disease.* London, 1914.

BROWNE (Sir T.). *Pseudodoxia Epidemica: or, Enquiries into very many received Tenets, and commonly presumed Truths.* London, 1646.

CAMPION (G. G.). *Elements in Thought and Emotion.* London, 1923.

—— "The Neural Substrata of Reflective Thought." *Brit. J. Med. Psychol.*, 1925, v, 65–82.

—— "The Organic Growth of the Concept as one of the Factors in Intelligence." *Brit. J. Psychol.*, 1928–1929, xix, 60–64.

—— "Meaning and Error." *J. Philosoph. Stud.*, April 1929.

—— "Thalamo-cortical Circulation of Neural Impulse ; New Integration of Thalamo-cortical Functioning." *Brit. J. Med. Psychol.*, 1929, ix, 203–217.

CLARK (W. E. LE G.). "The Structure and Connections of the Thalamus." *Brain*, 1932, lv, 406–470.

HART (B.). *Psychopathology; its Development and its Place in Medicine.* (Goulstonian Lectures.) Second edition, Edinburgh, 1929.

HEAD (Sir HENRY). *Studies in Neurology.* 2 vols. London, 1920.

—— *Aphasia and Kindred Disorders of Speech.* 2 vols. Cambridge, 1926.

HEAD (Sir HENRY) and HOLMES (G.). "Sensory Disturbances from Cerebral Lesions." *Brain*, 1911–1912, xxxiv, 102–254.

HORTON (LYDIARD H.). *Prince's 'Neurogram' Concept. Problems of Personality.* London and New York, 1925.

HUXLEY (T. H.). " On Sensation and the Unity of Structure of the Sensiferous Organs." *Nineteenth Century*, 1879, v, 597–611. Reprinted in : Foster (Sir M.) and Lankester (E. R.) (editors), *The Scientific Memoirs of Thomas Henry Huxley*. London, 1902, IV, 357–373.

JACKSON (J. HUGHLINGS). *Evolution and Dissolution of the Nervous System*. The Croonian Lectures delivered at the Royal College of Physicians, March 1884. London, 1884. (Reprinted from *Brit. Med. J.*)

JAMES (W.). *Principles of Psychology*. 2 vols. London, 1890.

——— *Psychology*. (Briefer course.) London, 1892.

——— *Some Problems of Philosophy*. London, 1911.

——— Quoted by S. Alexander, " The Artistry of Truth." *Hibbert J.*, Jan. 1925, p. 303.

McDOUGALL (W.). *An Outline of Abnormal Psychology*. London, 1926.

——— " The Confusion of the Concept." *J. Philosoph. Stud.*, Jan. 1929.

MITCHELL (T. W.). " Psychotherapeutics and Psychopathology." *Brit. Med. J.*, 1922, ii, 543–546.

MYERS (C. S.). " On the Nature of Mind." *Rep. Brit. Ass. Adv. Sc.*, 1931, London, 1932, xcix, 181–195.

PATTISON (A. S. PRINGLE-). Balfour Lectures on Realism. Third Series. London, 1933.

PIÉRON (H.). *Thought and the Brain*. Transl. by C. K. Ogden. London, 1927.

PRATT (J. B.). In : Drake (D.) (editor), *Essays in Critical Realism*. London, 1920, p. 97.

Problems of Personality. Studies presented to Dr. Morton Prince, Pioneer in American Psychopathology. London and New York, 1925.

RIVERS (W. H. R.). *Instinct and the Unconscious*. Cambridge, 1920.

ROBERTS (M.). *Warfare in the Human Body*. London, 1920. Chapter IV : " Inhibition and the Cardiac Vagus."

SANTAYANA (G.). *The Life of Reason*. New York, 1905. Vol. I : " Introduction, and Reason in Common Sense."

SEMON (R.). *Bewusstseinsvorgang und Gehirnprozess*. Wiesbaden, 1920.

——— *The Mneme*. London and New York, 1921.

——— *Mnemic Psychology*. London, 1923.

SHERRINGTON (Sir C. S.). " Some Aspects of Animal Mechanism."
    Rep. Brit. Ass. Adv. Sc., 1922, London, 1923, xc, 1–15.
—— *The Brain and its Mechanism.* The Rede Lecture, delivered
    before the University of Cambridge, Dec. 5, 1933. Cambridge,
    1933.
SMITH (Sir GRAFTON ELLIOT). " Notes upon the Natural Subdivision
    of the Cerebral Hemisphere." *J. Anat. and Physiol.*, 1900–
    1901, xxxv, 431–454.
—— *The Evolution of Man.* Second edition, Oxford, 1927.
—— " The New Vision." *Nature*, 1928, cxxi, 680–681.
—— " New Light on Vision." *Nature*, 1930, cxxv, 820–824.
—— *Human History.* Second edition, London, 1934.
SPEARMAN (C. E.). *The Nature of Intelligence and the Principles of
    Cognition.* London, 1923.
STOUT (G. F.). *The Groundwork of Psychology.* Revised by R. H.
    Thouless. Second edition, London, 1927.

INDEX

ABSTRACTION, neural mechanism involved in, 83

Action and thought, connection between, 38

— significance in mind-making, 38

Affective disposition of mind, 39

— elements entering every act of perception, how supplied, 76, 77

— factor, agent of organic growth of concept, 21

— — in consciousness, 109

— — in relation to concept, 104

— — inseparability of concept from, 21

— — names attached to, 21

— — processes, integration of, mechanism for, 23

— involving in circuit of neural impulse, hypothalamus, thalamus and cortex (*The Lonely Plough*), 135

— qualities total of all the senses influencing motor responses of the body, 36

— therapeutics in case of amnesia with disturbance of organic function, 129

Afferent nerve stimuli, in cerebrospinal nervous system, path taken by, 88

— — — site of redistribution, 88

Alexander, Prof. S., " Artistry of Truth " (quoted), 77

— correlation and identification of mental with neural processes, 14

— Gifford Lectures (1916 – 18), *Space, Time and Deity*, 1920, 49, 50 (note)

— identification of mental process with neural process, 50, 122

Amnesia, with disturbance of organic function, case of, 128

— — — origin discussed, 129, 130, 131

— — — — treatment, 129

Amphibian, most important change in, on emergence from fish-like ancestors, 19

Analysis and subsequent synthesis, Newtonian method of, future uses of indicated, 95

Analysis, psychological aspect of, 59

Anatomy, comparative, throwing light upon process of mental evolution, example of, 18

Animal, movements of, how consciously directed, 29

Anstie's principle, 118

Aphasia, 113, 114

— disability of, difficulties involved by, 55, 56

Apperceiving mass of Herbart, 9

Appetite, hypothalamus in relation to, 31

Appetites, function of, part of brain related to, 36

A priori data and sense data, commingling in acts of perception, 108

Aristotle, 7

Association areas, intercommunication of engrams through, 82

— — latest of, development in juxtaposition with cortico - motor areas, 111

— — of the cortex, 24

— — — — connexions established with, 23

— — See also *Cortical* association areas; *Thalamic* association areas

— fibres, 124

— of ideas, doctrine of, 64

Associationism in logic and psychology, demolition of, 50

Attention, focus of, 70, 71, 72

— — extended visual image in passing to fringe of consciousness, 72 (note), 73

— — neural correlate, 71, 89

— transference from concept to concept, 87, 88

BALFOUR Lectures on Realism (A. S. Pringle Pattison), (Trans-subjective inferences in Epistemology), 11

Bartlett, F. C., Types of Imagination (quoted), 120, and 120 (note)

Consciousness—*continued*
— conceptual correlate of active engram above level of, 86, 87
— — of latent engram below level of, 86
— datum of, 90
— fringe of, 72
— — extended visual image in, altering from focus of attention to, 72 (note), 73
— — neural correlate, 89
— interpenetration of, two aspects of, 103
— mental correlates of engrams below level of, 68
— method of finding and expressing attempted by W. James, 7
— multitude of engrams brought above threshold of, 89, 90
— passage of concepts into, 13
— relation to the brain (W. James), 5, 6
— states of, as subject-matter of psychology (W. James), 4
Corpus striatum, 29
— — activities of, how expressed, 30
— — translation of stimuli into action by, 34
Cortex, cerebral, activities of, influenced by hypothalamus, 23
— — affective organ of smell in primitive vertebrate, 35
— — and thalamus, neural impulses passing backwards and forwards between, 22
— — and thalami, neural paths connecting and functioning between, 116
— — anticipation of what might and did happen from past experience stored in (*The Lonely Plough*), 137
— — as storehouse of past impressions and experience, 130
— — — — character in *The Lonely Plough* illustrating, 135
— — connexion with mechanism in central nervous system concerned with muscular activities, 24
— — — with psychical functions in wounded soldier, 16
— — dominant part of in most primitive vertebrates, 35

Cortex, cerebral, fibre-connexions with cerebellum, 38
— — function of, 20
— — — in regard to sense of smell in animal, 34
— — — supreme, 35, 36
— — functions of, 27, 28
— — grouping of, multitudinous paths found in, 111
— — influencing involuntary muscles and secretions of ductless glands, 126
— — large part concerned with regulation of muscular functions, 38
— — linking of various parts of, 22
— — recapitulation of past experience stored in, excited by present surrounding (*The Lonely Plough*), 137-138
— — receptive instrument for impressions of smell, 33
— — seat of spacial projection and discrimination, 128
— — supragranular layer, dependence of mind on, 16
— — tonic control over function of thalami by means of cortico-thalamic paths, 116
— — transmission of fibres from thalamus to, 31, 32
— — — of neural impulses, to all parts of during thought, 112
Cortical association areas, 22, 123, 124
— — — activity of, illustrated, 110
— control, 92
— intercommunication tracts, 124
— motor areas, development of latest of association areas in juxtaposition with, 111
— phenomena, 116
Cortico-thalamic circulation. *See* Thalamo-cortical
— — (cortico-fugal), paths, 110, 116, 124
— — paths, function of, 78, 79, 107
Cytology, mental, 48

DATA, relevant, active selection of in process of perception, 10
Differential perception of visual sense-data, refinement in, 12
Disposition, cognitive, single constituent element of, 51

Eyes and hands, perfection in co-operation of, in attainment of manipulative skill and dexterity, 20

FACILITATION, establishment of engrammic systems by, 75

Fact, what is indispensable for complete knowledge of (W. James), 7

Facts, particular, nature of, 7, 8

Fibres leaving hemisphere, purpose and function of, 24

Fingers, skin of, acquiring heightened powers of tactile discrimination, 20

Flexor and extensor muscles, co-ordinated and simultaneous intensive adjustment of, neural potential supplying, 81

Food, pursuit of by dogfish, culmination of, how represented, 33

Fore-limbs, high specialization by flight in evolution of birds, 19

Forgetfulness, permanent, how resulting, 76

Freud, S., discoveries in psychology and psycho-pathology made by, 47

— illogical inferences of, 104

Froebel's school, 3

Functioning, lower and earlier levels of becoming active upon failure of higher levels, 121

GENERA and Species, query as to nature of, 83

Generalization, neural mechanism involved in, 83

Geniculate body, lateral, nature of impulses transmitted to by eyes, 35

Greek philosophers, view regarding knowledge of universals, 8

Growth-process of the concepts, how illustrated, 44, 45

HABIT and tradition, power of, in one individual, character in *The Lonely Plough* illustrating, 136

Hand and eyes, perfection in co-operation in attainment of manipulative skill and dexterity, 20

Hart, Bernard, affective therapeutics, 129

Harvey, William, discovery of the circulation of the blood by, when proved, 98

Head, Sir Henry, 2, 23, 86, 88, 114, 127

— *Aphasia and Kindred Disorders of Speech*, 56, 113, 114, 120

— central seat of consciousness, 107

— cortex as storehouse of past impressions and experience, 130

— essential organ of the thalamus, 20, 22, 37, 123

— investigation of sensation and the cerebral cortex, 15, 16

— neural schemata, 12

— part played by thalamus in sensation, 124

— researches on what is involved in tactile discrimination, 20

— *Studies in Neurology*, vol. ii (quoted), 111

— and Holmes (Gordon), on the essential thalamic organs, 109

— — function assigned to the essential organs of the thalami by, 76

— function of neural schemata, 70, 71, 105, 106

— — "Sensory Disturbances from Cerebral Lesions" (quoted), 68, 69, 82

Herbart, apperceiving mass of, 9

Hippocampal formation, dominant part of cerebral cortex in most primitive vertebrates, 35

— — efferent fibres from, 36

— — primitive, assumed function of, 36

Holme, Constance, *The Lonely Plough*, scene from exhibiting manifestations of neural processes in everyday life, 132 *et seq.*

Holmes, Gordon, 88

— central seat of consciousness, 107

— *See also* Head (Sir Henry)

Horton, L. H., Prince's Neurogram Concept (Studies in Personality, 1925), 149

Hudson, W. H., revival of lost memories during illness, 120

Hume, D., doctrine of association of ideas, 64

INDEX

Humour, decline in, result of fecundity of language, 54, 55

Huxley, T. H., the metaphysical problem of problems, 62

— on metaphysical speculation and physical theory, 94

— on the psycho-neural problem, 94

— query as to nature of genera and species, 83

— on sensory operations, 94

Hypothalamus, 24

— essential instrument of emotional expression, 30

— function of, 36

— in relation to appetite, 31

— influencing activities of thalamus and cortex, 23

—← thalamus and cortex, circuits of neural impulse between keeping up alternations of inconsequent thought and speech (*The Lonely Plough*), 147

— — — — emotional outburst involving, exhibited by character in *The Lonely Plough*, 143

— — — interactions of, causing mental absorption, shown in character in *The Lonely Plough*, 148

— — — neural circuit involving, seen in character in *The Lonely Plough*, 135, 142

IDEAS, association of, 64

— Realm of (Plato), 7

Illumination, awareness of, primary functions of eyes connected with, 35

Illusion, human, how explained, 10

Illusions, outgrowing of, 11

— use of, 11

Incito-motor centres, 114

Inhibition, conditions to which the term is applied, 79

— nature of, 81, 91

— process of, wrong inferences regarding, 80

Intelligence, definition of (tentative and provisional), 49

Interest, affective, 103

JACKSON, J. Hughlings, 114

— Croonian Lectures on *The Evolution and Dissolution of the Nervous System* (quoted), 117, 118, 121

Jackson, doctrine of evolution of the nervous system, 110

James, William, 2, 47, 85

— altered views regarding problems of knowledge connected with psychology, 4

— discussion of states of mind in relation to brain states, 5, 6

— 'fringe of consciousness,' 72 (note)

— 'general law' of perception stated by, 11

— posthumous work on *Some Problems in Philosophy* (1911), 3, 4

— *Principles of Psychology* (1890), 4 (quoted), 64

— psychological law or theory anticipated by, 1

— psycho-neural problem, 62

— *Some Problems of Philosophy* (1911) (quoted), 7, 8, 51, 66 (quoted), 99, 100

— *Textbook of Psychology* (1892), 1, 4 (quoted), 51 (note), 93, 94 (quoted), 99, 101

— — — quoted (Mental atom theory), 65, 67

— traditional view of concept held by, 65, 66

— view regarding Universal-worship, 7

— views as to backward state of psychology (1892), 4

— — on conception (1890), compared with those on percept and concept (1911), 6, 7

Janet, on cause of dissociation, 131

Judgments, considered processes involved in, 84

— logical, immediate, neural processes involved in, 92

— neural correlates of, 83, 84

— translation into words, how effected, 111

KEITH, Sir Arthur, concept of the author regarding, 43

— — — — enlargement of, 44, 45, 52, 108

Knowledge, affective and discriminative, integration of functions concerned with, 31

— cognitive elements of, relation of thalamo-cortical circulation of neural impulse to, 122

— comprehensive theory of, 102

L